PANDEMIC, EVENT, AND THE IMMANENCE OF LIFE

This volume reflects on different regional and national experiences of the Covid 19 pandemic, with contributions from India, Thailand, Singapore, Australia, Italy, United States, and Canada.

This book draws upon a number of approaches but especially the works of Deleuze and Guattari, Agamben, Derrida, Foucault, Habermas, Latour, and Serres. It looks at the methodological aspects of treating the pandemic, focuses on laying out the posthuman condition of the event largely problematizing the immanence of life which affirms the transversal Deleuzian ethic of life, and extends the politics of life to the domain of immunology. Together, the authors make it apparent that the pandemic is a multifaceted event, or many different kinds of events – virological, informational, phenomenological, social, and discursive. The authors skilfully develop these different dimensions of the pandemic event and show the relations between them. These essays will enrich the reader's understanding of the pandemic and its effects, while demonstrating the depth and breadth of the resources that humanities scholarship can mobilize to help us understand such phenomena.

This volume will be useful to students of posthumanism, medical humanities, health communication, political communication, semiotics, literature, cultural theories, and major strains of thought from contemporary continental philosophy.

NY Manoj is currently assistant professor at Centre for Culture, Media and Governance, Jamia Millia Islamia, and visiting fellow at the Global Centre for Technology in Humanities, Kyung Hee University, South Korea. He is the founding general secretary of Deleuze and Guattari Studies in India Collective, which has already organized six international conferences and numerous workshops on Deleuze and Guattari in India and the convener of the World Congress on Deleuze and Guattari 2020 held in New Delhi. Formerly a fellow at Centro Incontri Umani Ascona, Switzerland, currently he is associated with an international research project on critical postmedia studies in Asia in collaboration with Teikyo University, Japan and Kyung Hee University, South Korea. He is the coeditor of the books titled *Deleuze, Guattari and India: Exploring a Post-Post Colonial Multiplicity* (Routledge 2022) and *Deleuze, Guattari and the Schizoanalysis of Postmedia* (Bloomsbury, London 2023).

Saima Saeed is professor at the Centre for Culture, Media and Governance (CCMG) and foreign students' advisor, Jamia Millia Islamia, New Delhi. Published in well-known journals including *Journalism Studies, Society and Culture in South Asia, and Economic and Political Weekly,* she is the author of *Screening the Public Sphere: Media and Democracy in India* (Routledge 2013). She has been project director of major research projects funded by Indian Council of Social Science Research (ICSSR) and the University Grants Commission (UGC) and has earlier served as the media coordinator of JMI. Prior to joining academia, she has worked in leading news channels based in New Delhi. Her research interests include journalism and news studies, media and democracy, media and the margins, and history of media technologies and cultures.

Paul Patton is the Hongyi chair professor of Philosophy, Wuhan University, and Emeritus professor of philosophy at The University of New South Wales, Australia. He is a fellow of the Australian Academy of the Humanities and has served on the Council of the Australasian Association of Philosophy and the Executive Committee of the Australasian Society for Continental Philosophy. He has published widely on Deleuze and other continental philosophers and translated Deleuze's *Difference and Repetition*. He is the author of *Deleuze and the Political* (Routledge, 2000) and *Deleuzean Concepts: Philosophy, Colonization, Politics* (Stanford 2010).

PANDEMIC, EVENT, AND THE IMMANENCE OF LIFE

Critical Reflections on Covid-19

Edited by NY Manoj, Saima Saeed and Paul Patton

Routledge
Taylor & Francis Group
LONDON AND NEW YORK

Designed cover image: Getty Images

First published 2025
by Routledge
4 Park Square, Milton Park, Abingdon, Oxon OX14 4RN

and by Routledge

605 Third Avenue, New York, NY 10158

Routledge is an imprint of the Taylor & Francis Group, an informa business

British Library Cataloguing-in-Publication Data
A catalogue record for this book is available from the British Library

ISBN: 978-1-032-56481-4 (hbk)
ISBN: 978-1-032-83103-9 (pbk)
ISBN: 978-1-003-50778-9 (ebk)

DOI: 10.4324/9781003507789

Typeset in Sabon
by SPi Technologies India Pvt Ltd (Straive)

In the memory of those who have lost their lives to the Covid-19 pandemic

CONTENTS

CONTRIBUTORS

Daniela Angelucci is associate professor of aesthetics at University Roma Tre and co-director of the postgraduate course Environmental Humanities at University Roma Tre. She has been a member of the Presidency Board of Italian Society of Aesthetics. She is a member of the Scientific Committee of the review *La Deleuziana* and managing editor of the review *Lebenswelt. Aesthetics and philosophy of experience*. In 2016 she organized in Rome the 9th Deleuze Studies International Conference and Deleuze Studies Camp. Recent books and editions include *Filosofia del cinema*, 2013; *Deleuze and the concepts of cinema*, 2014; *Editions: Philosophical Essays on Nespolo's Art and Cinema* (with D. Dal Sasso), 2018; and *Deleuze in Italy*, 2019.

David R. Cole is the founder of the Institute of Interdisciplinary Research into the Anthropocene: https://iiraorg.com/. David is a philosopher of education and author, having produced more than one hundred significant publications and 15 books. He believes that the problematics of the Anthropocene can only be approached through collective practice and thought. Firstly, the complex dynamics that are at play need to be understood and rethought beyond limiting assumptions. Secondly, this exploration has to be translated to practical action on the ground that can be followed by communities. David works as an associate professor in education at Western Sydney University, Australia.

Gary Genosko is professor of communication and digital media at Ontario Tech University. He is a leading English language interpreter of the work of Félix Guattari. His books include *The Reinvention of Social Practices: Essays* *on Félix Guattari* (2018), (with Jay Hetrick) *Machinic Eros: Félix Guattari's Writings on Japan* (2015), and *Félix Guattari: A Critical Introduction* (2009).

Gregg Lambert is dean's professor of the humanities at Syracuse University, USA. He is author of many works of contemporary philosophy. In addition to *'The World is Gone': Philosophy in Light of the Pandemic* (University of Minnesota Press, 2022), from which portions of this chapter are taken, he is author of *'The People Are Missing': On Minor Literature Today* (University of Nebraska Press, 2021), and *Toward a Geopolitical Image of Thought* (Edinburgh University Press, 2021).

Sebastian Hsien-Hao Liao is distinguished professor of english and comparative literature at National Taiwan University. He received his PhD from Stanford University and was a postdoctoral fellow at Harvard University. In addition to being chief editor for three important literary journals in Taiwan, he also served as president of the Comparative Literature Association of Taiwan (ROC). His research interests include among others comparative poetics, Lacan, Deleuze and new materialism, modern Taiwan literature and culture, the Chinese diaspora, *Hongloumeng* studies, Taoist aesthetics, creativity studies, and cultural policy formation. He is currently working on three book projects: "Subjectivity in Taiwan Film", "The Alternative China", and "Deleuze and Taoism".

NY Manoj is currently assistant professor at Centre for Culture, Media and Governance, Jamia Millia Islamia and visiting fellow at the *Global Centre for Technology in Humanities*, Kyung Hee University, South Korea. He is the founding general secretary of the Deleuze and Guattari Studies in India Collective, which has already organized six international conferences and numerous workshops on Deleuze and Guattari in India and is also the convener of the World Congress on Deleuze and Guattari 2020 held in New Delhi. Formerly a fellow at Centro Incontri Umani Ascona, Switzerland, currently he is associated with an international research project on critical postmedia studies in Asia in collaboration with Teikyo University, Japan and Kyung Hee University, South Korea. He is the co-editor of the books titled *Deleuze, Guattari and India: Exploring a Post-Post Colonial Multiplicity* (Routledge 2022) and *Deleuze, Guattari and the Schizoanalysis of Postmedia* (Bloomsbury, London 2023).

Paul Patton is the Hongyi chair professor of philosophy, Wuhan University, and emeritus professor of philosophy at The University of New South Wales, Australia. He is a fellow of the Australian Academy of the Humanities and has served on the Council of the Australasian Association of Philosophy and the Executive Committee of the Australasian Society for Continental

Philosophy. He has published widely on Deleuze and other continental philosophers and translated Deleuze's *Difference and Repetition*. He is the author of *Deleuze and the Political* (Routledge, 2000) and *Deleuzean Concepts: Philosophy, Colonization*, Politics (Stanford 2010).

Saima Saeed is professor at the Centre for Culture, Media and Governance (CCMG) and foreign students' advisor, Jamia Millia Islamia, New Delhi. Published in well-known journals including *Journalism Studies, Society and Culture in South Asia* and *Economic and Political Weekly*, she is the author of *Screening the Public Sphere: Media and Democracy in India* (Routledge 2013). She has been project director of major research projects funded by the Indian Council of Social Science Research (ICSSR) and the University Grants Commission (UGC) and has earlier served as the media coordinator of JMI. Prior to joining academia, she has worked in leading news channels based in New Delhi. Her research interests include journalism and news studies, media and democracy, media and the margins, and history of media technologies and cultures.

Tony See is a visiting lecturer in the Nanyang Technological University (NTU) and the National Institute of Education (NIE) in Singapore. His research interest is in continental philosophy and comparative East–West philosophy. He is the author of *Community without Identity: The Ontology and Politics of Heidegger* (Atropos, 2009). He is appointed as research scholar in Osaka University in Japan (2016), and he is co-editor for the edited volume *Deleuze and Buddhism* (Palgrave, 2017). His most recent book is *The Wisdom of the Lotus Sutra: A Philosophical Exposition* (Palgrave, 2023).

Kenneth Surin is emeritus professor of critical theory at Duke University, USA. In addition to books and articles in theology and the philosophy of religion, he has published articles on political economy, political philosophy, French and German philosophy, the philosophy of art, the philosophy of education, sports and philosophy, the philosophy of literature, and cultural anthropology. His is the author of *Freedom Not Yet: Liberation and the Next World Order* (2009) and *Collected Essays on Deleuze and Guattari* (2019). He trained initially as an analytical philosopher and has published widely on the philosophy of Deleuze and Guattari.

Janell Watson is professor of French at Virginia Tech University, USA. She is author two books, *Literature and Material Culture from Balzac to Proust* and *Guattari's Diagrammatic Thought*, as well as many articles and chapters on literature, culture, and critical theory. She is editor of *The Minnesota Review: A Journal of Creative and Critical Writing*.

ACKNOWLEDGEMENTS

The idea of the book emerged amidst the tumult of a crisis that had virtually slowed down the whole world and inducted a new modality of administering life and death – the Covid 19 pandemic. The editors and contributors to this volume came together in the middle of the crisis to deliberate on the epistemic uncertainty that the event induced that beckoned a philosophical introspection. The essays meticulously curated here are mostly drawn from the online international lecture series titled 'On the Threshold of a Global Change (?): Pandemic and the Immanence of Life' that the editors convened during the pandemic. This volume features essay from the writers based in India, China, Singapore, Taiwan, Italy, Canada, Australia, and the United States.

As editors of the volume, we are grateful to everyone who contributed immensely to bringing this volume to fruition. The list is a long one. We are indebted to Jamia Millia Islamia for allowing us to organize this lecture series and making it a part of the centenary events of Jamia Millia Islamia (founded in 1920). Thanks are due to our colleagues Ian Buchanan, George Varghese K, Daniel Smith, Alex Taek-Gwang Lee, and Joff PN Bradley, who helped us in organising the lecture series and Indu Jain for her support. Also, to Gregg Lambert and Minnesota University Press for permission to use his paper. From the publisher's side, Shoma Choudhury and Shloka Chauhan extended immense support in the preparation of the volume, for which we are extremely thankful.

Portions of "Living in a World Without Others" were originally published in *The World Is Gone: Philosophy in Light of the Pandemic* by Gregg Lambert. Published by the University of Minnesota Press, 2021. *The World Is Gone* is licensed under a Creative Commons Attribution-NonCommercial-ShareAlike 4.0 International License (CC BY-NC-SA 4.0). Used by permission.

1

INTRODUCTION

Paul Patton, NY Manoj, and Saima Saeed

The Covid-19 pandemic appears to be over even though the virus is not going away. The best we can hope for is that it mutates into less lethal strains that are more infectious and therefore likely to supplant the spread of lethal varieties but that still confer sufficient immunity to protect those infected from reinfection for a time. There is reason to believe that the Omicron varieties meet these conditions and that the SARS-CoV-2 virus is being absorbed into the ecosystem of human pathogens in the same way that influenza became normalized after the 1918–1920 pandemic. Whether that is the end of the story remains to be seen, but it does now seem feasible to examine this extraordinary episode and to ask not only what happened and at what cost, but what has changed and what new possibilities for life have appeared in the aftermath. This is a daunting task given the complexity of a pandemic that encompasses so many different phenomena and levels of experience that it is difficult to comprehend as a single event. The virological, social, economic, political, and geopolitical dimensions of the pandemic, and their entanglements and ramifications, suggest it is more appropriately thought of as an array or assemblage of different kinds of event.

The attempt to describe the pandemic as an *event*, in the terms that this concept has been developed by Deleuze, Derrida, Foucault, Agamben, and others, has been a common thread running through many analyses of the pandemic.[1] As individuals and populations whose lives have been disrupted, rerouted, and governed by Covid-19, we are acutely aware of the multidimensional character of the pandemic event. As well as the physiological effects of the virus, we have experienced the effects on psychological well-being that result from extreme disruptions to established patterns of work and social life, including isolation from family members and social networks.

DOI: 10.4324/9781003507789-1

The policy responses to the pandemic in turn led to severe economic and social consequences, including unemployment for many. The proliferation of information and misinformation about the virus, its origins, and the effects of preventative measures such as vaccination, masks, and social distancing in turn exacerbated existing political divisions.

It is not only the complexity of the pandemic that makes it a problem for thought but also its contradictory character. On many levels, the pandemic confronted us with irreconcilable demands. Preserving the life of the population has long been a primary function of modern government, as has maintaining the social and institutional conditions in which the market economy can flourish. The quarantine measures introduced to control the spread of the SARS-COV-2 virus directly contradicted the needs of the economy. Similarly, the measures introduced to protect the lives of the elderly and those most exposed to the threat of lethal illness were incompatible with the quality of life of the younger and more healthy sections of the population. The spread of disease is at once both an intensely social and public phenomenon and, under quarantine conditions, an intensely personal and private experience. The governmental responses to the pandemic in many cases involved an unprecedented level of intrusion into the everyday lives of citizens, while at the same time the disruption of established patterns of work and social life led to new forms of social engagement and solidarity. These and other tensions at the heart of responses to the pandemic make it an especially forceful provocation to thought. As Deleuze suggests, it is not the familiar or that which we recognize that makes us think but the unfamiliar or dissonant object of an encounter.[2] An event as complex and disruptive as the Covid-19 pandemic is a powerful stimulus to thought, and not only in the medical and biological sciences. This volume brings together an international assortment of authors from humanities disciplines, some influenced by Deleuze and Guattari, but all of whom are driven to reflect on diverse aspects of the pandemic, its management, and its effects.

Questions of ontology and method provide the focus of essays in the first section of this collection. How should we begin to analyze a phenomenon as complex as this virological, informational, phenomenological, social, architectural, and discursive event? What should be the primary objects of this analysis, and in what frame of reference should we approach the pandemic? NY Manoj's 'Pandemic and the Question of Life: Towards a Posthuman Ontology' argues that the pandemic needs to be understood as a minor skirmish in a much wider revolution of our understanding of life and the human. On one level, it should be understood against the background of the emerging bioeconomy and the new biopolitical framework that it entails, resonant with but ultimately irreducible to Foucaultian biopolitics. On another level, it should be understood in the context of a critique of the implicit humanism in the prevailing discourse of the Anthropocene. Drawing on the work of

Donna Haraway, Claire Colebrook, Timothy Morton, and others, Manoj argues that the 'species thinking' embodied in the notion of the *anthropocene* may be considered a new variant of the paradoxical figure of man whose emergence and immanent demise Foucault analysed in *The Order of Things*. Finally, combining the vantage point of Deleuze and Guattari's assemblage philosophy and the symbiosis theory of life forms developed by Lynn Margulis, he argues for a new, posthumanist ontology of life that 'destabilises anthropocentrism and which, at the same time, resists the capitalist interventions of the bioeconomy' (35). On this approach, the pandemic can be seen as an indicator of our current condition, one that calls for a posthuman ontology and multispecies ecology that can affirm the multiplicity of life and resist its commoditization. The chapter ends with the rhetorical retort against the humanism latent in the theoretical discourses of Anthropocene offered by Foucault: 'to those who are still caught up with the warped and twisted forms of anthropologised reflections, "we can answer only with a philosophical laugh – which means to certain extent, a silent one"' (xx).

The construction of models was one of the important tools employed to govern the pandemic. Our experience of the pandemic was conditioned by the interaction and intersection of the variety of models deployed by governments in their efforts to moderate the impact of the disease on the health of populations, economies, and of course their own political fortunes. Against this background, Gary Genosko's 'Metamodeling the Pandemic: A Guattarian Approach' argues for the utility of Félix Guattari's concept of 'metamodeling' as a response to the forms of subjectivation produced by the measures supposed to govern Covid-19 and its impact on populations. Guattari does not propose a philosophy of modeling in the natural or social sciences but rather a critical approach to the deployment of models with the aim of encouraging self-organization or self-modeling. The schizoanalysis developed in collaboration with Deleuze is a form of metamodeling and, as Guattari suggests, it poses only one question: 'how does one model oneself?'[3] Thus, contrary to what the term suggests, metamodeling is not a higher-order practice of modeling models. It is rather

> a critical approach to method that prioritizes the construction of diagrams in auto-modelizations, that is, self-engendering cartographies of subjectivation, with neither hard pre-existent nor final determinations, but with analytic relevance to processes of singularization.
>
> *(41)*

Guattari's appeal to the agency of individuals and groups in the face of new forms of social surveillance and control reminds us that the disruptions occasioned by the pandemic are also potential sources for the emergence of new forms of social life, spaces of freedom made possible by new ways of working, communicating, or engaging with others: 'Metamodelisation scouts out points of rupture in dominant significations that can radically remake how a rapidly covidized subjectivity can auto-model itself' (xx).

Kenneth Surin's 'The Covid-19 Pandemic and Medico-Cyber-Political Discourse', lays out some of the theoretical apparatus that he suggests is needed to analyse the 'medico-cyber-political assemblage' that has emerged in response to the pandemic. Focused on 'mapping the terrain' of the discursive elements of this assemblage, Surin identifies Deleuze and Guattari's analysis of concepts, Hjelmslev's semiotics, and concepts derived from fuzzy logic as helpful theoretical tools. Importantly, he attributes to Deleuze and Guattari a 'narrative' understanding of concepts that abandons the traditional distinction between the concept and the particular intuitions that it encompasses in favour of a conception of concepts as particular interventions in a given field of reference. Hjelmslev's distinction between the deictic, connotative, and demonstrative functions of signs helps to develop an understanding of concepts as signs that create particular worlds. Surin points to the distinction drawn from fuzzy logic between, one the one hand, ambivalence between precisely determined states of affairs and, on the other, vague states of affairs, such as a 'heap' of things. He argues that this distinction is useful in identifying the constitutive vagueness of concepts drawn from epidemiology that are widely employed in discussions of Covid-19 and its effects, such as reproduction rates and fatalities. Together, these theoretical tools help us to see the novelty of the discourse that is neither a representation nor an expression but rather a constitutive element of the pandemic.

The final essay of the first section, Daniela Angelucci's 'Living Bodies and Uncanny Events', explores the now familiar idea that the pandemic should be understood as an event in the sense that Deleuze describes this in *Logic of Sense*. She begins with a meticulous analysis of the ways in which the SARS-CoV-2 virus exemplifies key elements of the uncanny as Freud defines it: at once both familiar and unfamiliar, inside and outside us, alive and not alive as are all viruses insofar as they are unable to reproduce themselves independently of the occupation of a host body, which is itself often destroyed by the viral infection. Her aim is not to pursue a psychoanalytic interpretation of the pandemic but rather to introduce Deleuze's description of events in the terms of a Stoic materialism that does away with dualism and transcendence and proposes that events are the incorporeal accompaniments of encounters between bodies. Angelucci argues that, by distinguishing the encounter and intermixture of bodies as bare physical 'happenings' from the incorporeal events that accompany them, Deleuze presents us with a materialist view of the world in which meaning nonetheless has a place, namely the peculiar nonplace of the incorporeal event that is inseparable from the encounters between bodies 'as the fog rising from a prairie is inseparable' (71). The Covid-19 pandemic is not only an exemplary expression of Deleuze's 'thought of immanence' but also a reminder of the unsustainability of ideas about the separation and hierarchy of species (73). 'We form a rhizome with our viruses, or rather our viruses cause us to form a rhizome with other animals' (73).

The second section of this collection comprises chapters that address the politics of the pandemic, where this includes both the ways in which it was managed and put to use by powerful political agents and also the political lessons that might be drawn from it, in the broadest sense of the term 'politics' that includes human relations to nature as well as the relations between communities and between individuals.

Saima Saeed's 'COVID-19 and the Production of Knowledge: Communication, Control, and the Citizenry' approaches the pandemic from the perspective of its representation in the public sphere, through the variety of informational mechanisms that form, preform, and perform the occurrence of a pandemic. With reference to theorists as diverse as Weber and Badiou, Saeed points to the incapacity of contemporary news media to adequately represent an epidemiological event as complex as the emergence, transmission, and mutation of a novel virus. In addition to the epistemological limitations of journalism and news media in dealing with events of this nature, the reality of the pandemic was further obscured by the actions of governments, pharmaceutical multinationals, and other political agencies who manipulated the facts and the figures involved for their own ends, chiefly the development of new forms of control over populations and the expansion of 'surveillance capitalism' that enhanced the profits of wealthy individuals and corporations at the expense of the poor and the vulnerable:

> the altered governance practiced and witnessed during the COVID-19 pandemic was marked by an unprecedented corroboration between the State, pharmaceutical giants and technologies of surveillance refurbishing networks of control managed by an infodemic that sold the pandemic to the world's population.
>
> *(90)*

The combined effect of this corroboration was a more or less organized misrepresentation of the pandemic that overran a public sphere that could no longer function as a site of resistance but only serve to reinforce what Deleuze described as mechanisms for the control of populations.

Tony See Sin Heng's 'Philosophy and Pandemics: Agamben, Deleuze, and Zoepolitics in an Age of Covid-19' explores the political impact of the pandemic. He presents Agamben's theoretical reflections on biopower and the role of the 'state of exception' as a means to understand how the pandemic served above all to legitimate a momentous extension of state power. Agamben's own commentary on government responses to the pandemic confirms this application of his earlier analyses of the sense in which politics in the West has always been a biopolitics. See takes Deleuze and Guattari's focus on the question of desire and the libidinal underpinnings of political movements to point to a possible development of biopolitical analysis, posing the question whether we might envisage a schizoanalysis of biopolitics that asks, for example, why people

> quietly accept state paradigms that view them as 'population' and 'statistics' instead of viewing them as citizens with rights? Why do they believe with all their heart and all their might that surveillance technologies and movement controls are the way to go? Why do people focus exclusively on vaccines as the solution to the coronavirus instead of other options?
>
> *(105)*

Finally, he asks whether the pandemic might not serve to redirect our political imagination away from biopolitics towards a 'politics of life as *zoe*'. Inverting the terms of Agamben's thesis about the switch from *zoe* to *bios* in Western political thought, he suggests that perhaps it is time 'to start asking ourselves whether we have had enough of biopolitics and whether there is still time to desire a *zoepolitics*' (105).

Sebastian Hsien-Hao Liao's 'Of Virus and Man: Wound, the Non-human, and Counter-actualization' proposes to rethink the human–virus relationship along lines suggested by Deleuze's philosophy of the event and the associated phenomenon of the wound inspired by ancient Stoicism. In a wide-ranging discussion, he applies to our current experience of the virus the stoic injunction adopted by Deleuze: how to become worthy of the events that befall us? In this light, the pandemic can be understood both as an extreme instance of human lack of control over the natural environment and an opportunity to recalibrate our relationship to that environment:

> *Amor fati* allows us to look our incorporeal wound in the eye and realize that we are never complete and insular subjects and always live symbiotically with other creatures and objects. This pandemic serves as a timely reminder and warning of human transgressions of the boundaries that should not have been transgressed.
>
> *(117–118)*

As such a reminder, the pandemic offers an opportunity to learn or to relearn how to live in nature as natural beings. It points to the possibility of avoiding the pathologies that stem from efforts to redirect the course of nature in a manner ultimately incompatible with the Tao of nature itself. For Liao, this is one way to understand what Deleuze means by recovering the capacity to 'believe in the world as it is', where the world is taken to be a process or movement in constant becoming. This implies rediscovering the capacity to undergo if not initiate change and the emergence of new ways of being.

The essays in the third section of this collection provide examples of the ways in which the pandemic has proved to be a stimulus to thought across the humanities. In some cases, this involves the creation of new concepts with which to understand ourselves and our time. In other cases, it places the experience of the pandemic in relation to other cultural phenomena in ways that enlarge or transform our understanding of both. Thus, Gregg Lambert's 'Living in a World Without Others' undertakes an existential reflection on the condition of many during and after the pandemic, namely isolation or living alone in a world without other people. His chapter is an early draft of part of what is now a published book, *The World Is Gone*.[4] In the essay published here, Lambert examines the condition created or exacerbated by the pandemic, namely to be condemned to an isolated existence as though marooned on an island in the manner of Defoe's Robinson Crusoe. He explores this condition through a close examination of Michel Tournier's retelling of Defoe's story *Friday*, originally published in 1967 as *Vendredi ou les limbes du Pacifique*, along with Gilles Deleuze's 1967 essay, 'Michel Tournier and the world without others', which reappears in revised form as an appendix to his *Logic of Sense* (1969). Following Tournier, Lambert outlines the destructive consequences for human subjectivity of living, literally, in a world without other people. Following Deleuze, he further explores the role of the 'other structure' in the creation of worlds and shows how his essay on Tournier's novel is an extraordinary analysis of perversion that inverts the usual terms brought to bear on this phenomenon: the pervert is not the one incapable of recognizing others, but rather a product of the absence of an 'other structure' that enables others to appear.

David Cole's chapter, 'The Dithering Pandemic', elaborates a concept of 'dithering' that he adapts from Kim Stanley Robinson's science fiction novel *2312*. Robinson represents the present age from the perspective of future historians who regard it as a moment of dithering in which human societies showed themselves incapable of acting in accordance with climate science to address the looming catastrophe. Cole calls for a 'philosophy of dithering' as a means to think the current circumstance of the Covid-19 pandemic as it unfolds in context of the Anthropocene. He fills out the concept with reference to Deleuze's concept of the 'stuttering' inherent in the truly creative writer's use of language, Deleuze and Guattari's concept of machines that function only in breaking down, Bataille's and Nick Land's respective versions of 'base' and 'libidinal' materialism, and the concept of the simulacrum developed in different ways by Deleuze, Pierre Klossowski, and Jean Baudrillard. His purpose in doing so is not simply to indicate the disorder and dysfunction of the present historical moment but also to suggest some ways in which it offers both the hope and the means towards another world. Guattari's concept of metamodeling discussed by Gary Genosko makes a brief appearance at the end of Cole's chapter, where it is introduced as a means to understand the hypercomplexity of societal functioning. For Cole, as for Genosko, metamodeling points to the ever-present possibility of escape from existing structures of social order, a possibility that is premised on the conception of society as 'a metamorphic system, with plans within plans, and lines of escape and digression wrought into its very functioning and thought' (156).

Finally, Janell Watson's 'Quarantine or Feast? Hospitality and the State of Plague' examines the reactions to Covid-19 through the lens of Michel Serres's reading of ancient Roman ritual and religion. She divides the public responses to the pandemic into those that impose quarantine and those that advocate modern analogues to the Roman ritual banquets intended to ward off the plague. The ambivalence reflected in these divergent social responses is present in the very concept of hospitality, which refers to the host who can be either guest or enemy, and in the pandemic considered as the modern equivalent of the state of plague that exemplifies 'the equivalence of hostility and hospitality' (166). Against the contemporary defenders of state authoritarian intervention such as Badiou, she defends Serres's embrace of the uncertainty injected into social life by the virus and his call for a 'politics of care predicated on absolute hospitality' (161). This ambivalence reaches into the nature of the social contract which, for thinkers such as Hobbes, is supposed to provide the foundations of the modern state:

> The open feast models a new social contract, under which humans live together, bound by the meal rather than by hostility toward a common enemy, as was the case with social bonds maintained in the state of war. *(168)*

Watson's wide-ranging discussion of Serres's work presents his diagnosis of the modern world as built on an authoritarian rather than a hospitable conception of reason, in which hostility and the domination of nature take precedence over hospitality and care for the world. For Serres, the history of myth, culture, and religion offers a better guide to the modern world, which can be understood as a new version of the ancient distinction between the world of the gods and that of its human underlabourers. The pandemic highlights the distance between these two classes, the differential social effects of quarantine, and the vast differences in the healthcare available to rich and poor.

Taken together, the essays in this collection explore some of the consequences of the different kinds of event – virological, informational, phenomenological, social, architectural, and discursive – that make up the pandemic event. They examine different dimensions of this complex event and point to the relations between them, thereby enriching our understanding of the pandemic and its effects. Beyond that, they take the pandemic event as a provocation to thought about our present psychic, social, political, and environmental condition, drawing attention to some of the ways in which this disruptive event helps us to perceive other modalities of living, both alongside other people and in nature more broadly understood. They demonstrate the depth and breadth of the resources that humanities scholarship can mobilize to help us understand the impact of a complex and world-changing phenomena such as the Covid-19 pandemic.

Notes

1 See for example Jemima Repo and Hannah Richter, 2022, 'An Evental Pandemic: Thinking the COVID-19 "Event" with Deleuze and Foucault,' *Distinktion: Journal of Social Theory*, 23: 2–3, 220–237; Paul Patton, 2022, 'In What Sense Is the Corona Phenomenon *political*?', in Pegah Mossleh (ed), *Corona Phenomenon. Philosophical and Political Questions*, Leiden and Boston: Brill, 125–132.
2 See *Difference and Repetition*, chapter 3, pp. 182–184 in the 2014 Bloomsbury edition.
3 Félix Guattari, 1996, *The Guattari Reader* (p. 132), ed. Gary Genosko, Oxford: Blackwell.
4 Gregg Lambert, 2021, *The World Is Gone: Philosophy in Light of the Pandemic*. Minnesota University Press.

PART I

Analysing the Pandemic

Ontology and Method

2

PANDEMIC AND THE QUESTION OF LIFE

Towards a Posthuman Ontology

NY Manoj

Introduction

This chapter is not an attempt to analyse the Covid-19 pandemic but to analyse the biopolitical imaginary which emerges through the governance and manipulation of 'life' in contemporary times using Covid-19 pandemic as the reference point. Life emerges as the ontopolitical object in the context of the emerging bioeconomy that draws its inspiration from the molecularization of life and the concomitant commodification that puts it into the global flow of markets and organ banks. This ontopolitics of life capitalises on the venture capital that assigns the biovalue to life, brings in a complex ecology of biopolitics, and redefines the notion of life in cultural, political, and ethical terms. The commodification of life is not relegated merely to the realm of species but to the molecular level which includes cells, genes and tissues. It is against this backdrop that the politics of pandemics should be deciphered. A pandemic is an instance of crisis which opens up hitherto unattended concerns regarding life. Combatting the Covid-19 pandemic was often portrayed as a crusade against the microbial beings using the vocabulary of war.

This chapter attempts to tackle the politics and commoditisation of life by resorting to a posthuman/nonhuman ontology and multispecies ecology. The chapter has three sections – the first deals with the imminent politics of life and the consequences of the new inquiries regarding the threshold of life. In the second section, this is further corroborated by the critique of anthropocentrism and the implicit revival of anthropos in the guise of species thinking in the discourse of the Anthropocene. This lays the foundation for a posthuman ontology. The third section focuses on the multiplicity of life by exploring the symbiotic relationships that sustain life, thereby challenging the

DOI: 10.4324/9781003507789-3

notion of 'individual' and 'species' as dominant categories of classification. It attempts to look at symbiosis as a Deleuzo-Guattarian assemblage and argues, following Deleuze and Guattari, that symbiotic relations have always been there in history. Finally, the paper argues for a posthuman ontology that questions the arborescent model of biology and can address the transversal multispecies connections that affirm the immanence of life withstanding its commoditisation by venture capital.

I

Pandemic and the politics of life

The Covid-19 pandemic is suggestive of the myriad ways in which the Foucauldian notion of biopolitics played out and, at the same time, marked the revival of various disciplinary machines of earlier epidemics, for example quarantine as a method of confinement. Instead of accepting this claim, we should refine the argument: the pandemic situation is a state of exception when the normalised forms of monitoring and surveillance by means of statistics and population profiles become more explicit. Apart from the normal register of biopolitics, we have witnessed an exceptional employment of various organisational forms – like that of the public health centres, quasi-judicial bodies for effective surveillance with the power to levy fines on people – and the 'becoming' of the decentralised modes of governance as effective surveillance machines. The emergency plan designed for the epidemic diseases in early Europe as summarised by Stuart Elden (2002) resonates with most of the health measures adopted during the Covid-19 pandemic.

It is quite interesting to note that the various measures of dealing with epidemics in early European society in all their crude forms were repeated in postcolonial India. The confinement of people to their homes, the patrolling by the police and otherwise constituted quasi-judiciary forms of power, and the declaration of certain streets or areas as Covid-infected wards which solicited more restriction and close surveillance are a few measures which resonated with the earlier modes of surveillance in European society. In *Madness and Civilisation* (2006), Foucault talks about the great confinement as a strategy of exclusion to contain leprosy. These strategies of exclusion were kept intact, whereas the role of the leper was later replaced by the poor, vagrants, prisoners, and the alienated (Foucault 2006: 6).

There was a marked difference in the exclusionary politics that unfolded during the spread of leprosy versus the strategy of governance employed against the plague. During leprosy there was an explicit exclusion of lepers with the marking of their bodies by hanging a bell around their necks, while the plague, because of its contagious nature, required confinement: 'it was not exclusion but quarantine … Not rejection but inclusion' (Foucault 2007: 45).

The streets of this confinement were controlled and policed based on the principle of surveillance through close and meticulous observation (*quadrillage*). This apparatus of surveillance which involved multiple separations was to ensure compliance to the rules and sustain the defined norm of health. The difference between the two epidemics was in the depth of the surveillance and control employed with an intensification of power.

In short, the plague strategy gave rise to the disciplinary diagrams. Though many of these disciplinary modes were apparent during the Covid-19 pandemic across the world, the politics of the pandemic exceed this frame and necessitate a post-Foucauldian framework of biopolitics characterised by the fusion of living and technological systems, especially in the context of bio-digital convergence.

This transition from the confines of the disciplinary society to the self-modulatory expanse of the societies of control is pithily captured in the small piece 'Postscript on the Societies of Control' written by Deleuze (1992). The transition from the society of sovereignty, via the disciplinary, to the control society is marked by the technological devices of simple machines, thermodynamic machines, and computers, respectively. All of these machines express social forms which embody the conditions for generating and using them. The disciplinary society is thus marked by the spaces of enclosure which are very clearly demarcated from the society ordered in time and distributed in space, whereas the society of control is a self-modulating space which has no exteriority. To find a space outside the self-modulating spaces of control or being imperceptible is almost impossible because of the fluid structure of the ever-evolving apparatuses of capture. Nail (2016) in his analysis finds the notions of control and biopower as synonymous in their form and content by resorting to the later lectures of Deleuze on Foucault. It is either that 'Deleuze makes explicit the idea of control implicit in Foucault's concept of Biopower or Foucault makes explicit the idea of biopower in Burrough's concept of control' (Nail 2016: 261). Though there are concepts that Deleuze develops from Foucault, say the diagram, the politics of life in the societies of control goes even further in positing a bioeconomy in the context of 'Nano-Bio-Info-Cogno' (NBIC) technologies. Deleuze foresaw the domination of codes in the new paradigm where individuals are fractured into data, codes, and passwords and exist as no more than masses, samples, data, and banks. The bio-informational paradigm, which is a blending of viral biology and information science, substantiates or perhaps even surpasses the Deleuzian notion of control.

These new objects – genes, atoms, bytes – have radically reconfigured the ontology of humans and the epistemic structure of the disciplines. The new sciences have dismembered the human body into organs, fluids, and codes. We have reached a stage in which perhaps a new body can be re-assembled from an organ bank of body fluids and genetic software or 'wetware'. The bio-genetic, neural, and mediatic information, which informs the process of life mining, becomes the new capital. Cognitive capitalism employs different methods to monitor the capacities of bio-mediated bodies like DNA testing, brain fingerprinting, neural imaging, body heat detection, and iris/hand recognition – all of which could be employed as surveillance techniques as well.

The Human Genome Project is at pains to unify the whole of humanity under the master sign of the gene, creating a new 'pan-humanity'. But the genetic unification project extends to the animal world too, thereby creating an inter-species web that enfolds all living matter in the universe. The sexual, racial, and natural differences which were the boundary-markers of a classical humanism have disappeared into the miasma of the posthuman, marked by disjunctive synthesis and transversal subjectivity. The autopoietic, self-organising capacity of nature is not confined to the human species alone, but to all living matter, driven by informational codes which interact in multiple ways with the social, psychic, and ecological environments. This complex field of data flows and information has resulted in a posthuman relational subjectivity which itself is a cumulative effect of all these forces. The informational power of living matter becomes the target of this new mode of capitalism which sees 'life as surplus' and which employs a different demography from that of Foucauldian biopolitics.

The question of life has been rearticulated in the domain of biopolitics and an emergent posthuman ecology focused on the chimeric and transversal connection between the life sciences and digital ecology. It is argued that bioeconomy has been a pertinent policy topic in the last decade, as it has been an important concern for the US National Science Foundation (Peters et al. 2023: 252). Taking a cue from the Foucauldian discourse of biopolitics, there has been a surge of concepts related to the *bios* which is indicative of the emerging bioeconomy – the new form of capitalism at the interstices of bio-scientific knowledge and biotechnologies. To cite a few: biovalue, which is referred to as the surplus value of vitality and instrumental knowledge that can be placed at the disposal of the human subject (Waldby 2000: 19), bioeconomics (Nicholas Rose 2001), biocapital (Sunder Rajan 2006: 2012), biocitizenship (Rose and Novas 2004), biowealth (van Dooren 2007), biosubjectivities (Wahlberg 2007), biosubject (Gerlach et al. 2011), bio-object (Niki Vermeulen et al. 2012), bio-knowledge (Petersen 2013), and bio-commodification (Dawson 2013).

Birch and Tyfield question the fetishisation of bio-objects and the apolitical attempt of STS scholars to address the new shift in the terms of modern capitalism without due concern given to the 'transformation of economic and financial process in modern capitalism' (2012: 301). The shift from the Foucauldian understanding of biopolitics to the new liberal eugenics of the new bioeconomy has been identified by Nicholas Rose (2007), who argues that the age of biopolitics is no more. Braun puts it in clearer terms that the difference between the two can be seen as 'the difference between state-led programmes that in the past sought to produce a particular population with particular traits and capabilities, and the ethical decision of the individuals in the present, who are exercising their choices in reproductive matters' (2007: 11). The new molecular biopolitics is not restricted to the state-led biopolitics of the individual and the population but is based on the consumer's individual reproductive choice and extends to cells, genes, molecules, and the genome. The bioeconomy is not based on morbidity and mortality as defined in terms of traditional biopolitics; rather it is anchored on vitality within an ethos of hope. The bio-objects like tissues, cells, and genes are disentangled from the material corporeality of the body and inducted into the network of technologies deployed in the biotech industry. The 'separable, exchangeable and reincorporable body parts' (Rabinow 1999: 95) are inducted into the global flow of markets and organ banks to create biovalue out of the yield of vitality.

These biosciences are no longer connected to the discourse of the truth and are calibrated to the interests of venture capital which unify the research being done in universities and the monopoly capitalism of patents. The stem cell, which can be transformed potentially into diverse sorts of cells, has been identified as a curious object among these bio-objects because of its pluripotent nature. The bioeconomy is based on the speculative hopes of biological potency that 'is often (mis)taken to be a primordial ontology upon which biocapitalism merely elaborates' (Helmreich 2008: 464). As Melinda Cooper (2008: 19) argues, 'life becomes literally annexed within the capitalist process of accumulation' and thus, we have the notion of 'life as surplus'.

The new biology emergent from molecular rescaling creates a new assemblage which redefines capitalist practices, colonial thinking (in terms of people from India volunteering for clinical trials which are outsourced from the US), as well as offering new permutations of subjectification at the genomic level. Thus, the realm of biopolitics which capitalises life at the molecular level opens up the possibilities of a new politics of life itself, which creates inescapable biopolitical bondage as well as the reconstitution of what we think of as 'life' in scientific, cultural, and ethical terms. The emerging bio-economy points to innovations in the scientific and technological realms and posits a biotechnological transformation of life and hence extension of the boundaries of life itself. The new possibilities of merging biological life and computation in the disciplines of bioinformatics and biocomputing become the ground for the emergence of this new economy based on life. There is an intricate similarity here: the basic forms of cellular life entail a complex structure akin to the computational one in their reiterative molecular processes which perform logical operations. Here the question is, as Eugene Thacker put it:

> the philosophical question of "what is a body?" is, in biotech, indelibly tied to the technical question "how is a body made?" or, more accurately, "what is a biomolecular body capable of? and how can that be enhanced?"

> Theories of biological life (the common trope of the "genetic code") are intimately connected to practices of engineering, programming and design – for instance, in how the genetic code in a test tube is implemented in online genomic databases
>
> *(Thacker 2004: 2)*

The new sciences unfold the computational aspects of the biological in terms of informational storage and replication in DNA, RNA, and multiple cells – the biologising of the digital in terms of using DNA as the substrate for new computing hardware, in resolving difficult computational problems, and in positing, for example, organic computers using organic memory technologies. This synergy of biological and computational systems is explicit in recent advancements like artificial neural networks, evolutionary computing, organic computing, mathematical biology, digital organisms, and so on. As Gillings et al. (2016: 180, 188) argue, 'the potential symbiosis between biological and digital information will reach a critical point … the biological and digital will become more integrated in the future … might become a symbiosis that coevolves through natural and artificial selection'. The advancement implied here is from the digitisation of biology to the synthesis of life from codes, and it seeks the possibility of artificial life.

The notion of bioeconomy is not posited as merely an outcome of technological and scientific advancements, it is constituted in the larger context of the incumbent reconfiguration of the relations between biology, informational science and nanotechnology, global climate crises, and the discourse of sustainable development which can aid in terraforming the planet as inhabitable. The policy discourse of the Organisation for Economic Cooperation and Development (OECD) and the European Commission posits this new economy based on the vitality of life, in the context of decarbonising the economy and becoming a climate-neutral continent by 2050 (European Commission 2020: OECD 2009). The OECD explains bioeconomy as 'the aggregate set of economic operations in a society that use the latent value incumbent in biological products and processes to capture new growth and welfare benefits of citizens and nations' (as quoted in Birch & Tyfield 2012: 300).

Thus, it is argued that the new economic paradigm, which is based on the disruptive power of the emergent biotechnology, is focused on the replacement of the linear fossil-fuels- and carbon-intense-products-based paradigm with a new range of renewable bioproducts. These technological convergences and emergent knowledge economies, while extending the limits of life, posit a new form of collective management of life, a new biopolitics. The molecular reordering of life cannot be simply divorced from the clutches of biocapitalism and biopolitical practices' optimisation of life. This new order of life is enmeshed in rights and patents, as multinational corporations own the patents of new species with the emergence of biopharming.

This posits a new muddled politics of life, which is further complicated with the 'becoming' of state as the techno-state, and it necessitates a new form of bioethics and an advanced awareness of the implied biopolitics. The pandemic should be placed in the context of this emergent bioeconomy, the analysis of which will not fit into the structure of a Foucauldian biopolitics, although we find some resonances here and there. What is required is an immanent politics of life and a posthuman ethics of life. As we have already seen how contemporary biopolitics employs and manages life in terms of the new political and social assemblages, now we will look into the epistemic inquiries which broaden the threshold of life in its micro and macro aspects.

Extreme Life: Life at the Edges

Jami Weinstein and Claire Colebrook (2017: 2), in their postulation of critical life studies, argue for the envisioning of a 'thoroughgoing interrogation of life' as it forms 'the most immediate of the political imperatives' in the current discourse of the extinction of life. The critical attitude is further explained in terms of a post-Kantian critical project notwithstanding its humanising tendency in unearthing the conditions in which life has been thought and constructed epistemically, not eliding the usage of life in terms of biopolitical measures, and in using life as a means to 'humanize, racialize, gender, pathologize, and manage human and nonhuman bodies' (2017: 2). This critical project of life marks a departure from the earlier problematisation of life in abandoning the conception of life as the ground which opens up the biopolitical field and the uncritical positing of 'life itself' as such, though some of them, especially Foucauldian inquiry, share the post-Kantian framework of critical inquiry.

Adding to these issues concerning life is the profound problem of the historicity of life and the humanist constraints put on the limits of life. It was in the modern episteme, according to the order of knowledge laid out by Foucault in *The Order of Things* (1970), that the representational taxonomic table of classical natural history was replaced by the notion of life, which marked the birth of modern biology. The movement was from the representational structure in terms of identities and differences into the interiority of life, thus construing life as the object of biological inquiry. Recent advancements in the study on life extend the limits of inquiry on life to both the molecular and planetary scales. According to Stefan Helmreich (2016: 1), the consolidated object of biological enquiry, the 'life itself' which was constituted around 1800, underwent an epistemic and material transfiguration to 'genes and cells' as the new objects of inquiry which are 'rearrange[d] and disperse[d], and exist in distributed laboratory choreographies that have them frozen, amplified, and exchanged'. Helmreich identifies three new domains in which the threshold of life has been extended to its vitalist edges in such a way that life forms and forms of life 'inform, transform and deform one another' (2016: 3). These limit biologies – artificial intelligence, extreme marine biology, and astrobiology – are suggestive of the post-biological threshold which defers the definition of life and reinterprets the biologistic framework of *bios*. Artificial life is not just a technological simulation of life, but a synthesis of new life in cyberspace and robotics, which are decoupled from fossil fuels and supersede organic life. Thus, the notion of life becomes a formalised account which can be transposed across media to 'include not just life-as-we- know-it, but also life-as-it-could-be' (2016: 5).

The genomic reshuffling of bio-matter and the digital representation and simulation of life in terms of biocomputing and bioinformatics destabilise the ontological foundation of life provided by organic life forms. In bioinformatics, DNA is rendered fully digital, and computational technology is used to model biology, whereas in the case of biocomputing, DNA is fully biological and rendered as computational in itself. Here the relation between biology and computation is inscribed in such a way that biology is available for computational processes like archiving, searching, editing, and pattern making, and biology becomes amenable to computation processes. This relation cannot be rendered in terms of hybridisation of the biological body and machine, or the definition of technology as a tool or as a means to an end. This interaction conjures a qualitatively different notion of the biological which is optimised or mediated by technology where the 'biological and the digital inhere in each other' (Thacker 2004: 7). This sort of a bio-mediated body or biomedia is a specific mode of organisation of matter corresponding to the control society, rather than a disciplinary society, where codes and passwords dismember the self-contained notions of subject, self, and organism. In short, this construal of the bio-mediated body exposes the informational substrate of bodily matter or matter's capability of being in-formational – pointing to a post-biological threshold at the heart of the discourse on 'life itself' – by reconfiguring the biological body in computational terms while keeping the biological materiality intact. Helmreich (2016: 8) puts it concisely: 'life becomes abstractable, metaphysical, something can be ported across substrates … free floating form'.

The other form of the vitalist edges of life is unfolded through the identification of extremophiles (often bacteria or archaea), which can sustain extreme conditions of life, in the larger domain of the marine microbiological inquiry of life. The lateral gene transfer that happens among marine microbial beings which can sustain ecologies of extreme temperature, pressure, and chemistry questions the Darwinian arborescent natural classification of the tree of life and the pushing of the elementary biological form from the species to DNA. Microbial beings able to thrive in otherwise unnatural ecologies in deadly environments are referred to as extremophiles. Microbial beings which can survive in more than hundred-degree-Celsius hot springs and submarine hypothermal vents are referred to as hyperthermophiles, whereas the ones which survive in the extreme conditions of Antarctic ice are referred to as psychrophiles. The existence of barophiles (extreme conditions of pressure), halophiles (high concentration of salt), and acidophiles (very acidic environments) points to the artificial and relational division made by us on what is natural or unnatural in terms of life, and to the plasticity and flexibility of life which is yet to be mapped (Lopez-Garcia 2005). The numerical abundance (microbial biomass is almost one-third of earth's living biomass) (Kallmeyer et al. 2012) and taxonomic diversity of the microbial organisms, including the microbial eukaryotes in the ocean, enable them to play functional roles in terms of the chemical transformation process (including the symbiotic relation that they can have with larger organisms), the aggregate of which can be tangible at a planetary scale. This microbial diversity brings in a problem of classification, as species and population cannot be a unit of analysis as far as the microbial world is concerned.

The construal of diversity into species, which is the unit of biological classification, runs into philosophical problems as it is not possible to identify these species based on observable morphological traits because of their microscopic size. So, speciation here is indirect, based on approaches which combine the genotypic, phenotypic, and phylogenetic properties. This is further corroborated by the complexity offered by the lateral gene transfer in microbes across and within the species and even domains, and the resorting to genes rather than record fossils to identify the deep genealogy which blurs the genealogical relationships and phylogeny, and question the Darwinian representational structure of knowledge about the history of life. As Helmreich argues (2016: 9), there can be 'no universal phylogenetic tree of organisms based on such a reduction to genes' and the volume of gene transfer which is '20 million billion times per second in the oceans' disrupts the Darwinian notion of natural classification based on the lineages of descent. Furthermore, the notion of asexual, many-directed connection instead of sexual reproduction implodes the stability of the categories relevant to the organisation of knowledge about the history of life on earth. The philosophical implication of these 'extreme metabolisms, jumbled genealogies and shifting scales' (Helmreich 2016: 11–12) lies in the emergence of genes representing the flow of life whose morphological similarities and differences are made corporeal by the infusion of computation via bioinformatic representation and the adoption of relation instead of unity as the parameter which destabilises the classificatory and representational ordering of knowledge of life. What is affirmed is the multiplicity of life in a Deleuzian sense.

If marine microbiology deals with the microbial domain of life, the domain of astrobiology is at the opposite pole of infinity, dealing with the notions of extraterrestrial life and cosmic life. These can be considered analogous to extremophiles, as the extremes of life here are caught up in a 'secularized supernatural; its orbits extend beyond and embrace our planet' (Helmreich 2016: 15), pushing its own limits. Reminiscent of the renaissance episteme and at the same time quite different from the Foucauldian ordering of knowledge in a simulational paradigm, this inquiry is about the traces of life, which can be called 'biosignatures', fingerprints of life, left behind by the extraterrestrial life. The traces that are left behind can be a direct signature, where the traces are evidence of organic molecules, or remote signatures, which can be about the spectral signature of life in extraterrestrial space. The signifier of life is caught up, in a deconstructive fashion, in the web of endless signifiers as it is constantly repositioned; and each framing of life could completely alter its definition.

In a sense, the notion of universal life remains not accessible, not to be deciphered, as a domain not yet known. As Helmreich (2016) argues, there can be a faith in forms and ultimately in life as these explorations are always operating at the edges of life. Thus, the three disciplines – artificial life, extreme marine microbiology, and astrobiology – deal with the limits of organic, earthly, and cosmic life. Everything organic and non-organic, along with the human and non-human, becomes unified under the logic of 'life', which is an infinite potential – as the reimagining of spaces of life only takes us to the immanence and multiplicity of life.

II

~~Anthropocene~~: Against the New Humanism

The pandemic event testifies to the interspecies entanglement and posthumanist ontology which dismantled the unrivalled position of human subjectivity situated at the heart of Western metaphysics. It also testifies to the impending crisis of the contemporary, the trouble with which we are living, that is the 'damaged planet' marked by environmental uncertainties, ocean acidification, loss of biodiversity, the extinction of species, global warming, climate change, and much more. The emerging discourse around the Anthropocene, though in its nascent stage, brings to the fore certain theoretical contradictions vis-á-vis the posthuman ontology and the notion of anthropos. Let us consider the philosophical problems that imploded the category of anthropos in the ordering of knowledge which laid the foundation for posthuman ontology. Here the detailed archaeological analysis of Foucault comes to our rescue in problematizing the notion of human by explicating the very condition of its emergence in the epistemic ordering of knowledge. In the light of the Foucauldian dismissal of the anthropos, this paper will address the implicit anthropocentrism in the discourse of the Anthropocene.

In Foucauldian archeological ordering of knowledge pertaining to the human sciences, man emerged as an epistemic concern only in the modern episteme. As Foucault (1970: 308) rightly points out, 'Man is a quite recent creature, a demiurge of knowledge fabricated with its own hand less than 200 years ago. He has grown old so quickly as he had been waiting for thousands of years in darkness for that moment of illumination in which he could be known'. There was no epistemological consciousness of man as such before. This means that before the end of the 18th century man did not exist any more than the potency of life, the fecundity of labour, and the density of language. It was in the modern episteme, as per the archaeological analysis of Foucault, that the modern theme of the individual who speaks, lives, and works emerges within the laws of philology, biology, and economics. To quote Foucault (1970: 316):

> if man's knowledge is finite, it is because he is trapped, without the possibility of liberation, within the positive contents of language, labour and life; and inversely if life, labour and language may be posited in their positivity, it is because knowledge has finite forms.

These limiting factors which constrain forms of knowledge also become fundamental criteria for the possibility of knowledge in the human sciences.

The epistemic configuration of man ran into serious philosophical issues, which question the validity of the human-centred approach. The emergence of man as an epistemological category is possible in the finite structure that precedes and moulds him – life, labour, and language. In the Kantian fashion these limiting structures which precede the human become the condition for the possibility of the human sciences to emerge in the modern episteme, facilitating the epistemological constitution of the human subject. Foucault terms this the 'analytic of finitude' as the positivities of finitude become the foundation for knowledge. It is in this fundamental-positive pair that we find 'the transcendental repeats the empirical, the cogito repeats the unthought, and the return of the origin repeats its retreat' (Foucault 1970: 315–316). Here man appears as a fact to be studied empirically and the same time becomes the transcendental condition for the possibility of all knowledge, complicated by the unthought which evades him constantly, while being preserved as the cogito which is the source of all intelligibility and the product of a receding history in its search of an origin, while being the foundation of that history.

Caught between the eschatological and positivist approaches, man was treated as an 'empirico-transcendental doublet' which attempted not to reduce one to the other. But the attempt to strike the balance between the empirical and transcendental approach in Merleau-Ponty also became a reductive project, in which 'the empirical, in man, made stand for the transcendental' (Foucault 1970: 321). This congenital problem is further complicated by the doubling of cogito and the unthought as a dimension of our reality, an otherness that cannot be grasped within the structure of pure consciousness. Here the dichotomy is between 'man as both an experiencing subject and the never fully understood object of that experience' (Gutting 1989: 203). Foucault argues that the transcendental ego put forward by Husserl is not the resolution of this doublet but an instantiation of 'man' as empirico-transcendental doublet, as any of these polarities failed to address the opaque unthought and thus harbour the tension between man as the transcendental subject and empirical object of study. The other doubling of the man in the modern episteme is that of cogito and the unthought which pure consciousness tries to grapple with. The unthought, argues Foucault, and the human are contemporaries at the archaeological level (Foucault 1970: 326), which cannot be completely assimilated into the structures of cogito. It unfolds the reality of man as an experiencing subject and the never fully understood object of that experience. It becomes the other of the man, which is 'not only a brother, but a twin, born, not of man, nor in man, but beside him and at the same time, in an identical newness, in an unavoidable duality' (Foucault 1970: 326). Thus, the modern cogito cannot affirm the being of man as the unthought always lies 'in itself and outside itself, at its borders yet also in its warp and woof'.

The final problematic which constitutes the doubling of Man is in terms of the notion of his origin, which is conceived as an 'ever elusive', 'a remoteness and a distance that constitutes him' (Foucault 1970: 336). This constant retreat of the origin, according to Foucault, is 'posited in the extreme recession of origin', a sort of primordial temporality which is ontologically distant from him. Thus in the existential logic man is doomed to pursue this fruitless project of seeking the loci of his being and thus he fails in his attempt to get back to his origin. The analytic of finitude is preserved at the core of this search for his essential being or historical origin, and this becomes the transcendental source of the constitution of history which is imagined ironically in the human consciousness. Any such empirical historical inquiry will have to evade the question of being or the origin. Thus, as Foucault argues, 'return is posited only in the extreme recession of origin' (Foucault 1970: 334). In this historical inquiry, Foucault identifies two strains, which either propose a total withdrawal or total return. In Hegel and Marx, the project of historical inquiry is oriented towards the future as the fulfilment of essential being, or identification of original truth which leads to the end of history. In contrast, the projects of Nietzsche and Heidegger constitute the question of origin or essence as a mere absence, which was present in the past. This absence can only be made sense of by becoming aware of what is being lost. The undue focus on the human, for Foucault, was nothing other than the new form of dogmatic slumber. Thus Foucault pronounced the death of the human (as an epistemic category), and it created a deep void which unfolds many potentialities and new possibilities. The future possibility of a non-human approach is thus articulated by Foucault unfolding the internal inconsistencies in the construal of anthropos as the central figure of epistemic engagement. It is against the backdrop of the Foucauldian critique of the subject and the anthropos that we will analyse the notion of Anthropocene, as delineated in the influential book by Dipesh Chakrabarty (2021).

The controversial figure of the anthropos, which was deemed to have suffered a philosophical death in the ordering of knowledge postulated by Foucault, is refurbished in the discourse of the Anthropocene. This revival is not a repetition of the same, but with a significant difference. The emergent category of the anthropos is constituted as a 'planetary geological agent' (Chakrabarty 2021: 31) in a transhumanist vein, as a 'geophysical force capable of changing, with fearsome consequences, the climate system of the planet as a whole' in unprecedented ways (Chakrabarty 2021: 3). It is not the individual subject which has a political agency as articulated in the human histories, but a collective and historical entity, a geological force, impacting the ecosystem and geochemistry in an unprecedented fashion and on a planetary scale. For Dipesh Chakrabarty (2021: 1), this epochal shift marks an 'awareness of the planet and its geobiological history' and also the birth of the planet as 'an emergent object-category of human concern'. He identifies a doubling of the figure of the human, as an epistemological problematic emergent in the scientific discourse on climate change within the domain of history – the 'human of the humano-centric history' and the human as the geological force which is not accessible to the humano-centric narratives of history. The contradiction between the planet and the globe, deep time and human time, the simultaneity of the long 'now' of the geological scale and the 'now' of human history, the difference between the 'globe' in global warming and globalisation is significant in the 'differently scaled chronologies' (Chakrabarty 2021: 15).

The stratigraphic registering of the new epoch of Anthropocene has sparked a lot of controversy as there are at least 80–90 alternatives to the notion of the Anthropocene (Chwałczyk 2020): Chthulucene (Haraway), Capitalocene (Moore), Plantationocene (Tsing), Technocene (Hornborg), Homogocene (Mann), Neganthropocene (Stiegler), and Eremocene (Wilson), to list a few. The differences are based on the speculative beginning of the Anthropocene. Paul Crutzen and Eugene Stoermer (2000) identify the beginning of the Anthropocene with the industrial revolution, specifically with the invention of the steam engine by James Watt, whereas Simon Lewis and Mark Maslin (2018) have dated it to the year 1610 and proposed the 'Orbis hypotheses' as the starting point. This controversial speculation about the beginning of the Anthropocene makes possible the different types of '-cenes', contributing to the multiple definitions of the Anthropocene.

Considering all of these confusions regarding the various interpretations of the Anthropocene, Chakrabarty put forth four theses regarding the methodological challenges posed to the rendering of history that relies on human experience. The anthropogenic explanation of climate change questions the age-old traditional difference between human history and natural history that characterised the discipline of history in the 19th and 20th centuries. Citing the major historians like Collingwood, EH Carr, Vico, and Croce, Chakrabarty (2021) elucidates how the foundational dimension of Western thought, the Hegel-inspired anthropocentrism especially in the domain of history, which construes the human as the biological agent, is undone with the climate change scientists' portrayal of humans as the geological agent. Though Braudel, with the notion of *long durée*, attributed agency to non-human entities like the climate, his rebellion was mitigated by the shared assumption of two temporalities attributed to human history and geological history, the latter of which takes a longer time to make significant changes and is thus not deemed as relevant in historiography.

Though the natural historians made the breach wider, they were also caught up in the conceptual analysis of humans as biological agents. The climate group researchers introduced the question of scale to conceive the human as a geological force, 'which runs and exceeds human time' (2021: 10). Here the onus is on the doubling of the figure of the human, pointing towards the reevaluation of humanist history and thus re-positing the human subject on a planetary scale as a geological agent. Though the humanist histories are rejected, the Anthropos is still retained in the structure by treating it as a geological agency and positing the doubled figure of the human as 'human-human' (traditional history) and 'non-human-human' (geological history). To quote Chakrabarty:

> we are left with three images of the human: the universalist-Enlightenment view of the human as potentially the same everywhere, the subject with capacity to bear and exercise rights; the postcolonial-postmodern view of the human as the same but endowed everywhere with what some scholars call "anthropological difference"—differences of class, sexuality, gender, history, and so on. This second view is what the literature on globalization underlines. And then comes the figure of the human in the age of the Anthropocene, the era when humans act as a geological force on the planet, changing its climate for millennia to come.
>
> *(Chakrabarty 2012: 1–2)*

The scientific discourse on climate change which posits the collective agency of the human subject in the age of Anthropocene poses some epistemic problems. While positing the human as a geological force, the subject attains neither the subject nor the object position in terms of the subject–object dichotomy that has plagued Western metaphysics. This becoming 'force' of the collective subjectivity of the *anthropos* reveals a philosophical problem – the collective subjective position as a species is experientially inaccessible while being cognitively accessible – which denies an ontological position to this collective subjectivity. In short, the planetary focus and temporal scales are not directly available to the phenomenological realm, while they continue to be the determining factors of our lives. In a Latourian fashion, Chakrabarty addresses this as a 'pure, non-ontological agency' (Chakrabarty 2012: 13). The following thesis on the Anthropocene elaborates the position of the merging of different time scales and the 'folding of the human into the air, the sea, the soil and the DNA' (Dibley 2012: 139), thereby necessitating a category to think through the crisis – a species thinking, a *long durée*, that can bring the 'planetary and the global, deep and recorded histories, species thinking and critique of capital' (Chakrabarty 2021: 37) together into the fold. The crisis in question reveals the relevance of the conditions for the existence of life and its intricate web of synergistic connections, which calls for the knowledge of the human as a species notwithstanding the 'postcolonial suspicion of the universal' (Chakrabarty 2021: 42). The new universal of the 'species', emerging from a shared sense of the crisis, is always subtracted from the myth of a global identity and calls for a new kind of cosmopolitanism, a negative universal history (Chakrabarty 2021: 47–48).

The concept of the Anthropocene opens up the temporal and spatial scale, to consider the 'humanoid influence in the molecular makeup of the biosphere, in planetary cycles of carbon, nitrogen, and phosphorus, in geological strata and rates of extinction' (Woods 2014: 133), which find the human species to be the active agent of the geological epoch 'over multiple and incommensurable scales at once' (Chakrabarty 2012: 1), coalescing the vast inner molecular space and trans-scalar entities like the hyperobjects of Timothy Morton (2013). The emergence of the scale critique as a reflexive and analytic category opens up the possibility for the conception of climate change, global warming, along with other natural calamities and disorders collectively as the epoch of the Anthropocene, thereby revisiting and questioning the notions of history, society, and technology to discern a non-human and broader history. But this very possibility can also function as the limits of knowledge. In a Kantian fashion, it becomes the transcendental condition for the creation of a knowledge system and discourse around the Anthropocene, reintroducing the once imploded and dismissed notion of the human subject – which is now geologically reinscribed – into the epistemic discourse.

It is quite pertinent to explore the tenability of the concept of the Anthropocene as a negative universal category (Chakrabarty 2021), which is claimed to be subtracted from being subsumed. The notion of the 'inclusive disjunction of the Anthropocene' (Colebrook 2016: 441) is a clue to understand the problematic in a Deleuzo-Guattarian perspective to overcome the 'either–or' mode of accepting either the unity of the human at the cost of posthumanist and post-colonialist positions, or the diffusion of the all-inclusive narrative at the cost of a specific interpretation of the Anthropocene. It is argued that the anthropogenic definition of the new stratification of the current geological phase generates a 'hyper humanism along with a hyper-moral reterritorialisation' (2016: 442) that is all too human. Though the concept of the Anthropocene deterritorialises the notion of the earth coded in a particular way, it reinscribes the previous modes of stratification and the various other humanities into its fold by subsuming them in its mode of abstraction, axiomaticisation, and exchange, and seeing it as either proto-Anthropocene or as its effect. The question is how to think beyond the reterritorialisation of everything into the fold of the Anthropocene, and the restoration of the earlier grand narratives with the consecration of the geologically inscribed universal subject. The focus should be on the ruptures and limits to escape from the codes of the Anthropocene and imagining forms of stratification free from the determinations of the Anthropocene *socius*. For Colebrook, it is an intensification of the concept of the Anthropocene to ask 'what other stratifications might be imagined after the Anthropocene ... to think of other planetary scales where organic life has no prima facie value' (2016: 442–443). It is about the possibility of positing a 'nonhuman minor mode of stratification' (2016: 443) beyond the singular scale of Anthropocene stratigraphy. To quote Colebrook from her criticism of the Anthropocene's adoption of singular geological time; 'if we read the earth in terms of geological strata, then we conclude that a species emerges, takes its toll on its own conditions of life, ends a certain mode of life and then humanity comes to a close' (Colebrook 2016: 443). This calls for a review of the notion of species history and the discourse of the human as a geological agent in the larger context of the stratigraphic thinking proposed by Deleuze and Guattari (1987).

To think of the Anthropocene in stratigraphic terms is to posit it as existing with divergent and incompossible non-anthropocentric worlds, instead of the one-dimensional perspective emerging from the geological reading of the earth, privileging the deep time of its discernible layers over others. Strata in a Deleuzian sense are like 'black holes' or 'occlusions striving to seize', which operate by coding and territorialisation, but the body without organs constantly escapes them and becomes deterritorialised. It is between the body without the organs and the strata that we find assemblages. For Deleuze and Guattari, 'the assemblage is between two layers, between two strata; on the one side it faces the strata ... but the other side faces something else, the body without organs or the plane of consistency' (1987: 40). The assemblage opens up the possibilities of deterritorialisation by virtue of being proximate with the forces which destabilise it. This proximity of various divergent and incompossible worlds opens up the proliferation of differences and questions the universal humanity articulated in terms of 'the species', which can be still considered as a terraformer of the passive earth. To quote Colebrook again,

> It is the case that there is a species that calls itself "man" and that discovers itself to be an agent of geological force; it is also the case that there is no such thing as "man", and that planet earth has sustained forms of life

> (human and nonhuman) that are not folded around a conception of universal humanity or species-being.
>
> *(2016: 443–444)*

Besides this, the stratification of the Anthropocene, apart from subsuming other ways of articulating the crisis, already anticipates a chronology (before and after in a linear fashion) which rules out the possibility of transversal connections and is caught up in the limited confines of the scales of geological stratification. However, in a Deleuzian sense, we should 'superimpose a thousand tiny Anthropocenes or all the lived and unlived potentialities of the earth' (Colebrook 2016: 449) in a stratigraphic manner. These large-scale transversal patterns of relation existing amongst ontologically unrelated domains question the transcendental tendency which is articulated in terms of the universal sign of species. Rather, the species should be considered as a terraforming assemblage, as this stratigraphic thinking can posit a new ethics and postulate a new people and a new earth. Thus, the notion of species which is already fraught in the domain of natural sciences re-merges in the convergence of the human caught up in geological time – the human reinscribed at the level of species and the human beleaguered with the moral charge of the despoliation. Though there are reasons for articulating the consecration of the figure of human in the Anthropocene, this reinstatement cannot be divorced completely from the charge of transcendence. As Timothy Morton puts it more cogently, 'Perhaps Ananthropocene would have been more like it or ~~*Anthropocene*~~' (Morton 2012: 231–232).

Taking the recent Covid-19 pandemic as an occasion for posing the questions regarding the crisis of the now, in this chapter so far we have discussed how the notion of life has been drastically redefined in terms of the new epistemic inquiries and the imminent politics built around it, and how the question of the anthropos and other limiting factors has shaped the positing of the Anthropocene. Here the pandemic is considered only as an instance of triggering the questions regarding the deep entanglements of life and the disavowal of the implied anthropocentrism present even in its critique. Now, in the concluding section we will focus on the multiplicity of life in the context of Deleuzo-Guattarian philosophy and its intersections with new biological research, especially the symbiosis thesis of Lynn Margulis.

III

Life and Multiplicity

In the discussion of recent epistemic inquiries redefining the notion of life and the critique of the notion of the Anthropocene, we have analysed the tenability of the concept of species, especially in the context of extending the threshold of our inquiries regarding the notion of life and in the context of species thinking in the Anthropocene. Here we explore the philosophical implications of the recent research in the domain of biology – the nucleic acid analysis like genome sequencing and high-throughput RNA techniques – which has pointed out the importance of the symbionts present in plant and animal species that are significantly functional in certain metabolic pathways and physiological functions. This has raised certain concerns regarding the notion of the biological individual and the centrality of the notion of species, and it asserts the multiplicity of life.

Deleuze and Guattari's notion of rhizome and assemblages becomes more important in the analysis of new developments in the domain of biology. Through a Deleuzo-Guattarian lens, the phenomenon of symbiosis can be considered a rhizomic assemblage which destabilises the hierarchical and representational 'tree' models of biology. This can be read as a move against the traditional biologists who reduced life to the notion of species, which is identified as a sharing of perceptual qualities of anatomy and physiology. As reiterated in the discourses of Anthropocene, the species emerge as a category with a longevity which can represent life from the beginning till its death, and hence the inscription of the human as species in that discourse. Various theories regarding life in the life sciences were epistemically limited to the domain of species thinking: Theodor Schwann's postulation of cell theory (constrained cells to the category of species), Mayr's postulation of species as concrete reproductive entities, and the variation and inheritance postulated by the reemergence of Mendelism and Morgan's genetics were all confined to the umbrella category of species despite its potential to breach the epistemic boundaries. It has been argued that even the data procured through DNA sequencing and Carl Woese's dissection of subunit ribosomal RNA was also epistemically placed to strengthen the arborescent classificatory system based on species existing in biology (Shostak and Lundy 2016: 17–18). Darwinian inquiry regarding the lineages of life also ended up only prioritising the premier quality of species in terms of competition. In the backdrop of this traditional classificatory system in biology, which reduces the notion of life to a taxonomical table and arborescent model, we should posit the notion of symbiosis and the Deleuzo-Guattarian theory of assemblages to envisage the multiplicity of life.

The recent innovations in the field of scientific inquiries facilitated by technological advancements have opened up a new microbial world, which could change our conceptions regarding the planet's biosphere. This microbial world pertains to cellular organisms which include prokaryotes (archaea and bacteria), the eukaryotic organisms like fungi, yeasts, algae, and protozoa, and non-cellular organisms like viruses, their replicable parts, and other derived materials like genomes, plasmids, and cDNA (OECD 2007: 59). The microbial diversity accounts for the numerical abundance, species abundance, and functional and taxonomic diversity to the point that the precise classification of the microbial world in terms of the traditional categories becomes difficult. The bacterial species alone, argues Dykhuizen (1998), account for 10^7 to 10^{12} variants, excluding microbial eukaryotes and archae, which together will be even more immense. The ecology of viruses is also vast, to the extent that only 3,700 species have been identified and classified, whereas it is estimated to be 10^5 to 10^{13} species and adding up to 10^{30} viruses in the biosphere. This significantly shows that microbial organisms constitute a significant share of the biomass and are integrated within planetary life (Suttle 2005).

It is not the microbial diversity alone, but how they are functionally integrated into life on the planet creating complex and intermingled relationships between micro and macro vectors of life is also very pertinent. Lynn Margulis, the proponent of the theory of symbiosis argues that the cellular mitochondria is the result of a synthesis that happened two billion years ago with a free-living bacterium, which she termed symbiogenesis. It is argued that all the individual living organisms are nothing but products of various symbiotic relations that they enter into with the microbial and non-microbial world. Thus, the eukaryotic cell is already an assemblage in the Deleuzo-Guattarian sense. It is argued that modern biological accounts of the singular and unified individual which are defined anatomically, embryologically, physiologically, genetically, and evolutionarily have become untenable as the 'individual' posited by these domains of life sciences is permeated and punctured by other species, especially the microbes (Gilbert et al.2012: 327–333). The healthy human adult is arguably host to trillions of bacteria, whereas the human gut has a symbiotic relationship with 150 species of bacteria and 1,000 major bacterial groups. Gilbert et al. (2012: 327) argues that 'the gene set contained by this symbiotic metagenome is 150 times larger than that of the human eukaryotic genome' and this excludes the 'symbionts of human airways, skin, mouth or reproductive orifices'. Lynn Margulis (1998: 122) argues against the monogenetic characterisation of individuals which is well exemplified in the case of the cow for whom 'microbes do the work of grass digestion' which otherwise is not digestible in the absence of cellulose-degrading microbes. She further claims that 'indeed the cellulose-degrading microbes, in a very real sense, are the cow'. In the same vein, she also asserts the vital role of another microbial inhabitant – the virus – which is otherwise portrayed as our enemy: 'viruses are no more germs or enemies than are bacteria and human and other cells, as they always have. Like bacterial symbionts, viruses are sources of evolutionary variation ... we are viruses' (Margulis 1998: 63–64). As a result of the work of Margulis and others, the genetic individuality which is anchored on sex and the inheritance of the chromosomal complement is being eclipsed by hereditary symbiosis, and thus microbial symbionts form the second type of genetic inheritance challenging the one genome/one organism of classical genetics (Gilbert et al. 2012: 330).

The genetic identity which supersedes all other identities has lost its position as the defining factor for the exemplification of unity and wholeness of any being at the level of the individual and the species (Dupree 2012) despite the recent developments in the field of genomics since 'our biology is being determined by the genes encoded in our DNA along with the genes of our microbial partners' (Blaser et al. 2013: 213). All of these point to the destabilisation of the units of taxonomy such as species and individual, as both appear to be chimerical in the light of the infiltration of microbial beings. This problem was articulated by Betsy Foxman and Mariana Rosenthal (2013: 200) when they claimed that 'our microbiota are ourselves: their genes are our genes and their functionings are our functionings'. What is asserted is aparallel evolution and veritable becoming, which is not at all teleological or conforming to the lines of descent and filiations. The rhizomic and the transversal relations established between the host and the symbionts scramble the genealogical trees.

The cultural drive against the microbial world as demonic is propagated by medical discourse, which conforms to the static taxonomic classification of orthodox biology and which precludes the possibility of symbiotic relations. The metaphysics of one and the many, and the question of identity and difference, are the metaphysical notions behind this drive towards the exclusion of microbes. Given these notions of symbiogenesis and symbiotic relations that define life and belie the notion of individuals and other identitarian categories like species, we need to go beyond the species thinking which is dominant in the discourses of Anthropocene. Deleuze and Guattari disavow the traditional philosophical postulation of 'one and the many', as it is a false choice. Instead, they privilege the notion of multiplicity which rejects the notion of the self-contained subject, any presupposed unity, and notion of a totality which are 'produced and appear in multiplicities' (Deleuze 2006: 310). The notion of the multiplicity of life should be posited against any attempt to essentialise life in terms of identity and difference. Symbiosis can be considered a Deleuzo-Guattarian assemblage as the part–whole relation articulated by assemblage never falls into the trap of holism or the aggregative theory of external relations. As Posteraro argues, the Deleuzo-Guattarian notion of assemblage can be effectively employed to make sense of contemporary research in the field of life sciences and the deterritorialised notion of individuals plagued by the invasion of microbes and evolving with them (2020: 402). In the Deleuzo-Guattarian assemblage the part is neither subsumed under the whole as it remains external to the relations that it enters into and the whole which is the assemblage itself. The parts maintain autonomy and individuality and hence the assemblage is not a mere integration of the parts. In the Deleuzo-Guattarian sense, Posteraro (2020) argues, the organism can be considered an assemblage which anticipates the holobiont, which is nothing but the integrated organism which 'comprises of both host and persistent populations of symbionts' (Gilbert et al. 2012: 327–28). The abstract machine, which is a reservoir of potentials and hence virtual, can anticipate some of the features of the hologenome, which is the collective genome. For Deleuze and Guattari, 'if evolution includes any veritable becomings, it is in the domain of symbiosis' (1987: 238) which 'spans kingdoms, dislocate[s] and propagate[s] genetic information across independent evolutionary lineages, afford[s] new capacities to otherwise less able individual organisms' (Posteraro 2020: 421). Thus, the organism is not merely an assemblage of organs but becomes part of a bigger assemblage which the organism plugs into. It is no more defined by the species or genre, organs, or functions; rather it is defined in terms of the assemblage it enters into.

Deleuze and Guattari didn't confine their theory of assemblage or symbiotic relationships to the domain of biology, as there has always been a symbiotic process in history which is evident in the principles of nomadology. It is never the filiations that are important here but 'alliances, alloys; these are not successions, lines of descent, but contagions, epidemics, the wind' (Deleuze and Parnet 1987: 69). Deleuze and Guattari give examples of rhizomatic connection between the baboon and the cat, the wasp and the orchid. In the first case, the virus has formed rhizomes between them, and in the latter case it is in the molecular or sub-molecular particle where the alliance occurs. The example of the man–horse–stirrup–weapon assemblage has changed the entire history of warfare and, thus, social history. This is a social form of animal–man symbiosis, which gives the knight optimum efficiency as the speed of the horse is interconnected with the stationary point of the lance and the stirrup which stations the knight on the moving horse. This new assemblage between man, animal, and weapon produces speeds and effects in the battlefield and is connected to other collective assemblages of enunciation in medieval literature. So, this assemblage is not a technological advancement; it can only be considered as 'a capture of code, surplus value of a code, an increase in valence, a veritable becoming' (Deleuze and Guattari 1987: 10). The technology is primarily social as it is the social machine that selects, assembles, and executes the technical machine. This horse–man–stirrup assemblage's function was related to the grant of land and the beneficiary's obligation to protect the domain from intruders in the age of feudalism. Thus, it is a social machine first and then a man–animal–technological assemblage. As Deleuze and Guattari (1987) note,

> the organic and the social machines are not formed in the same way they function, and the technical machines are not assembled in the same way they are used but imply precisely the specific conditions that separate their own production from their distinct product.

What is affirmed is the multiplicity of life, which becomes a welter of lines and forces. The affective qualities of the assemblage can challenge the classification based on groups, genera, and species as things which appear to be very disparate but that can come together, and those which are apparently similar but become dissimilar in the lines of effect that it produces in Spinozist terms. For example, the plough horse and the racehorse: though they belong to the same species, in terms of effect they are dissimilar as the plough horse has more similarity with the plough ox, whereas the racehorse has more affinity with the racecar in terms of the effect and assemblage that it generates. Thus, life is less defined in terms of the genus, species, organs, or functions; rather it is defined by the assemblage that it enters into.

Conclusion

In this paper the pandemic is considered an event which unfolds certain modes and vectors, and which prompts us to think about the implied politics of life. The molecular and the sub-molecular particles with which we are allied in terms of life create 'transversal communications between different lines' that 'scramble the genealogical trees' (Deleuze and Guattari 1987: 11). Microbes were not at all considered as major political actants, except for situations like a pandemic or an epidemic outbreak. They were mostly understood or studied in terms of the immunity and pathogens that can breach human immunity. What contributed to this kind of a strict division between the human environment and the virosphere or largely the realm of microbes is the metaphysical principle which underlies the conception of life in terms of 'one and the many' and identity subsuming the notion of differences. The study of metagenomics, which is the study of collective genomes, evinces the multispecies relationships and groupings which affirm the multiplicity and the rhizomic assemblage of life. Of course, the Covid-19 pandemic is a multispecies event as it is caused by a zoonotic virus that can traverse between human and nonhuman species. At the same time the Covid-19 pandemic is considered as an Anthropocene pandemic because it is caused by anthropogenic circumstances like climate change, deforestation, and so on. While addressing it as a result of the anthropogenic alterations in the biosphere, we need to think of a multispecies belonging which goes beyond the 'human exceptionalism and bounded individualism' that are the 'old saws of western philosophy' (Haraway 2016: 30).

Haraway urges us to stay with the trouble in the mixed, disturbing, and turbid time and 'to stir up, to make cloudy, to disturb' the existing framework of thought as the 'overflowing richness of biology' forces us to a sort of 'tentacular thinking' (Haraway 2016: 1). The task for her is to become capable 'to make kin in lines of inventive connections as a practice of learning to live and die well with each other in a thick present' (Haraway 2016). She posits the Chthulucene in disagreement with the notion of the Anthropocene as 'it is not about ongoingness ... species man doesn't make history ... and history must give way to geo stories' (2016: 49). The discourse on Anthropocene, for Haraway, relies on an 'unthinkable theory of relations, namely the old one of bounded utilitarian individualism' (Haraway 2016). The Chthulucene is 'earthy worlding' which is 'thoroughly terrain, muddled and mortal' which is imbued with the 'ongoing multispecies stories' (Haraway 2016: 55).

What we have encountered in this chapter is the centrality of 'life' in the contemporary discourse and how it emerges as an epistemic category which reconfigures the notions of life by extending it to unforeseen and unthinkable stretches. What we need is a new ontology of life which destabilises anthropocentrism and which, at the same time, resists the capitalist interventions of the bioeconomy. I would like to postulate a posthuman ontology of life. The relationality proposed by the posthuman subject transgresses the boundaries of species and questions the anthropocentric definition of life which results in the division of *Bios* and *Zoe*, which is the non-human vital force of life. This *Zoe*-centered egalitarianism which stands for generative vitality, argues Braidotti (2013), is the transversal force that binds the previously separated species and categories and is considered as an effective response to the opportunistic political economy of biogenetic capitalism to exploit from the commodification of transpecies. The discourse of Anthropocene, as we have seen, implicitly invokes humanism by reinscribing the human as a geological agent, and in the undue importance given to the species as a category. As Foucault (1970: 342–43) rightly points out, to those who are still caught up with warped and twisted forms of anthropologised reflections, 'we can answer only with a philosophical laugh – which means to a certain extent, a silent one'.

References

Birch, Kean and David Tyfield. 2012. 'Theorizing the Bioeconomy: Biovalue, Biocapital, Bioeconomics or…What?', *Science, Technology and Human Values*, 38(3): 299–327. https://doi.org/10.1177/0162243912442398

Blaser, Martin, Peer Bork, Claire Fraser, Rob Knight and Jun Wang. 2013. 'The microbiome explored: recent insights and future challenges', *Nature Reviews Microbiology*, 11: 213–217.

Braidotti, Rosi. 2013. *The Posthuman*. Cambridge: Polity Press.

Braun, Bruce. 2007. 'Biopolitics and Molecularization of Life', *Cultural Geographies*, 14: 6–28.

Chakrabarty, Dipesh. 2012. 'Postcolonial Studies in the Era of Climate Change', *New Literary History*, 43(1): 1–18. https://doi.org/10.1353/nlh.2012.0007

Chakrabarty, Dipesh. 2021. *The Climate of History in a Planetary Age*. Chicago and London: Chicago University Press.

Chwałczyk, Franciszek. 2020. 'Around the Anthropocene in Eighty Names: Considering the Urbanocene Proposition', *Sustainability*, 12(11): 4558. https://doi.org/10.3990/su12114458

Colebrook, Claire. 2016. "A Grandiose Time of Coexistence': Stratigraphy of the Anthropocene', *Deleuze Studies*, 10(4): 440–454. https://doi.org/10.3366/dls.2016.0238

Cooper, Melinda. 2008. *Life as Surplus: Biotechnology and Capitalism in the Neoliberal Era*. Seattle: University of Washington Press.
Crutzen, Paul J. and Eugene F. Stoermer. 2000. 'The Anthropocene,' *IGBP Newsletter*, 41(17): 17–18.
Dawson, Ashley. 2013. 'Biohazard: The Catastrophic Temporality of Green Capitalism', *Social Text*, 31(1): 63–81.
Deleuze, Gilles. 1992. 'Postscript on the Societies of Control', *October*, 59: 3–7.
Deleuze, Gilles. 2006. *The Fold: Leibniz and the Baroque*, Translated by Tom Conley. London: Continuum.
Deleuze, Gilles and Felix Guattari. 1987. *A Thousand Plateaus*. London: Continuum.
Deleuze, Gilles and Claire Parnet. 1987. *Dialogues*, Translated by Hugh Tomlinson and Barbara Habberjam. New York: Columbia University Press.
Dibley, Ben. 2012. 'The Shape of Things to Come: Seven Theses on the Anthropocene and Attachment', *Australian Humanities Review*, 52: 139–153.
Dupree, John. 2012. *Processes of Life: Essays in the Philosophy of Biology*. Oxford: Oxford University Press.
Dykhuizen, D.E. 1998. 'Santa Rosalia Revisited: Why Are There So Many Species of Bacteria?' *Antonievan Leeuwenhock*, 73(1): 25–33.
Elden, Stuart. 2002. 'Plague, Panopticon, Police', *Surveillance & Society*, 1(3): 240–253. https://doi.org/10.24908/ss.v1i3.3339
European Commission. 2020. *Proposal for a Regulation of the European Parliament and the Council Establishing the Framework for Achieving Climate Neutrality and Amending Regulation (EU) 2018/1999 (European Climate Law)*. Available at 52020PC0080 - EN - EUR-Lex. Accessed on 10 July 2023.
Foucault, Michel. 1970. *The Order of Things*. New York: Vintage Books.
Foucault, Michel. 2006. *Madness and Civilization*, Translated by J. Murphy and J. Khalifa, New York: Routledge.
Foucault, Michel. 2007. *Abnormal: Lectures at the College de France 1974–75*. London, New York: Palgrave.
Foxman, Betsy, and Mariana Rosenthal. 2013. 'Implications of Microbiome for Epidemiology', *American Journal of Epidemiology*, 177(3): 197–201.
Gerlach, N., Hamilton, S., Sullivan, R. and Walton, P. 2011. *Becoming Biosubjects: Bodies, Systems, Technologies*. Toronto: University of Toronto Press.
Gilbert, Scott F., Jan Sapp and Alfred I Tauber. 2012. 'A Symbiotic View of Life: We Have Never Been Individuals', *The Quarterly Review of Biology*, 87(4): 325–341.
Gillings, M. R., M. Hilbert and D. J. Kemp. 2016. 'Information in the Biosphere: Biological and Digital Worlds', *Trends in Ecology & Evolution*, 31(3): 180–189.
Gutting, Gary. 1989. *Michel Foucault's Archaeology of Scientific Reason*. Cambridge: Cambridge University Press.
Haraway, Donna. 2016. *Staying With the Troubles: Experimental Futures*. Durham, NC: Duke University Press.
Helmreich, Stefan. 2008. 'Species of Biocapital', *Science as Culture*, 17(4): 463–478.
Helmreich, Stefan. 2016. *Sounding the Limits of Life*. New Jersey: Princeton University Press.
Kallmeyer, J., Pockalny, R., R. Adhikari, D C Smith, and S. D'Hondt. 2012. 'Global Distribution of Microbial Abundance and Biomass in Subseafloor Sediment', *Proceedings of the National Academy of Sciences*, 109(40): 16213–16216.
Lewis, Simon and Mark Maslin. 2018. *The Human Planet: How We Created the Anthropocene*. London: Penguin Random House.

Lopez-Garcia, P. (2005). 'Extremophiles', in Muriel Gargaud, Bernard Barbier, Herve Martin and Jacques Reisse (eds), *Lectures in Astrobiology*, 657–679. Heidelberg: Springer.
Margulis, Lynn. (1998). *Symbiotic Planet*. New York: Basic Books.
Morton, Timothy. 2012. 'Ecology Without the Present', *Oxford Literary Review*, 34(2): 229–238.
Morton, Timothy. 2013. *Hyperobjects: Philosophy and Ecology After the End of the World*. Minneapolis: University of Minnesota Press.
Nail, Thomas. 2016. 'Biopower and Control', in Thomas Nail and Nicolas Morar (eds), *Between Deleuze and Foucault*, pp. 247–263. Edinburgh: Edinburgh University Press.
OECD. 2007. *OECD Best Practice Guidelines for Biological Resource Centres*. Paris: Organization for Economic Co-operation and Development. https://www.oecd.org/sti/emerging-tech/38777417.pdf
OECD. 2009. *The Bioeconomy to 2030: Designing a Policy Agenda*. Paris: Organisation for Economic Cooperation and Development. https://www.oecd.org/sti/emerging-tech/34823102.pdf
Peters, Michael A., Peetar Jandric and Sarah Haynes. 2023. 'Biodigital Technologies and the Bioeconomy: The Global Green Deal?', *Educational Philosophy and Theory*, 55(3): 251–260. https://doi.org/10.10180/00131857.2020.1861938
Petersen, Alan. 2013. 'From Bioethics to a Sociology of Bio-knowledge', *Social Science and Medicine*, 98: 264–270.
Posteraro, Tano. 2020. 'Assemblage Theory and the Two Poles of Organic Life', *Deleuze and Guattari Studies*, 14(3): 402–432. https://doi.org/10.3366/dlgs.2020.0410
Rabinow, Paul. 1999. *French DNA: Trouble in Purgatory*. Chicago: University of Chicago Press.
Rose, Nikolas. 2001. 'The Politics of Life Itself', *Theory, Culture and Society*, 18(6): 1–30.
Rose, Nikolas. 2007. *The Politics of Life Itself: Biomedicine, Power and Subjectivity in the Twenty-First Century*. Princeton: Princeton University Press.
Rose, Nikolas and Carlos Novas. 2004. 'Biological Citizenship', in Aihwa Ong and Stephen J. Collier (eds), *Global Assemblages: Technology, Politics, and Ethics as Anthropological Problems*, pp. 439–463. Oxford: Blackwell.
Shostak, Stanley and Marcia Lundy. 2016. 'Symbiogeny and the Rhizomatic', *Trends in Developmental Biology*, 9: 18–27.
Sunder Rajan, Kaushik. 2006. *Biocapital*. Durham: Duke University Press.
Sunder Rajan, Kaushik. (ed.). 2012. *Lively Capital*. Durham: Duke University Press
Suttle, Curtis A. 2005. 'Viruses in the Sea', *Nature*, 437(7057): 356–361.
Thacker, Eugene. 2004. *Biomedia*. Minneapolis: University of Minnesota Press.
Van Dooren, Thom. 2007. 'Terminated Seed: Death, Proprietary Kinship and the Production of (Bio)wealth', *Science as Culture*, 16(1): 71–93.
Vermeulen, Niki. Sakari Tamminen, and Andrew Webster (eds). 2012. *Bio-objects: Life in the 21st Century*. Farnham: Ashgate.
Wahlberg, Ayo. 2007. 'Measuring Progress: Calculating the Life of Nations', *Distinktion: Scandinavian Journal of Social Theory*, 14: 65–82.
Waldby, Catherine. 2000. *The Visible Human Project: Informatic Bodies and the Posthuman Medicine*. London: Routledge.

Weinstein, Jami and Claire Colebrook. 2017. 'Introduction: Critical Life Studies and the Problems of Inhuman Rites and Posthumous Life', in Jami Weinstein and Claire Colebrook (eds.), *Theorizing Beyond the Posthuman*, 1–14. New York: Columbia University Press.

Woods, Derek. 2014. 'Scale Critique of the Anthropocene', *Minnesota Review*, 83: 133–142.

3

METAMODELLING THE PANDEMIC

A Guattarian Approach

Gary Genosko

Before we bear down on where we have been for some time, among the waves of a global pandemic, with the phalanx of vaccines rolling out unevenly across the globe, I want to explain Guattari's (2013) sense of metamodelling that he deploys in his book *Schizoanalytic Cartographies*, and briefly discusses in several interviews. A few general observations are in order. Guattari does not have a fully developed theory of models, which one would find in philosophy of science, for example, in which the relationship between theory–model–world is elaborated and argued. He does not propose a model as such, although he refers to schizoanalysis as a metamodel, not a generally applicable model in the spirit of much of the work done in communication modelling in the 1950s, but in the spirit of omnidirectional critique of existing models. For Guattari takes up with metamodelling a productive and creative critical perspective on modelling, which he aims squarely at standardisation, normalisation, and uncritical visibility. Metamodelling is directly related to a practice which brings about the production of new subjectivities loosened from conformity and adequation to existing models in the spirit of an escape from normopathic capture into the future of new reference points for auto-management.

Guattari's overriding concern is with the production of subjectivity. Imagine what he would have said about Covid and governance by means of epidemiological models. Epidemic models inform planning at all levels of government for the implementation of strategies of control of infection, narrativised as 'flatten' as in reduce – or better 'plank the curve', as in reduce infections to zero – the curve that represents the incidence rate (usually an average over a few days), or at least to reduce the average number of persons one person infects to less than one (the reproduction or R number over time,

DOI: 10.4324/9781003507789-4

hence Rt), thus ending or slowing the forward transmission of the virus. As everyone now knows, in many constituencies this has been extremely difficult to accomplish for a number of reasons.

Models are, of course, imperfect; they are always selective simplifications of phenomena, and in this case it is hard to make even short-term forecasts with incomplete data and limited knowledge about the behaviour of the virus, which public health measures work best, the precise intensity of epidemic control measures, and where they are most needed at any given time. The categories of analysis are extremely broad (susceptible–infected–recovered or dead as in no longer transmitting) and strong–none–weak controls. Models of Covid behaviour are the 'revealing objects' of epidemiologists, to modify a term ('working objects') discussed by Mary S. Morgan (2012: 380), and they emerge from a long tradition of mathematical modelling, conceptual development, and principles of scientific visualisation within the field, with a few pertinent historical reference points in earlier pandemics (i.e., 1918 Spanish flu pandemic). They are the artefactual products of training, imagination, tinkering, modification, and ongoing debate. For instance, are we in a pandemic or a syndemic in which biomedical solutions like vaccines would be if used alone sorely inadequate to address the interconnected epidemics of socioeconomic inequality, racial injustice, and climate catastrophe (and conversely, the intimate relationship between racial and environmental justice)? Models manage, articulate, and manipulate content, and if their inferential scope is greater than an extreme event they will have achieved 'abstract typicality' (Morgan 2012: 389), hence applicability would extend beyond the novel coronavirus to other such viruses like SARS and MERS, H1N1, and maybe further. This balance between particularity (too much granularity) and generality (not enough granularity) is usually hard won over time and is often clearer in retrospect.

There is a contiguous relationship in Guattari's thought between all forms of signification and power. This is not, as far as I am aware, of much concern to philosophers of science concerned with models. It is, however, the perspective of a Guattarian metamodeller interested in the ways in which collective subjectivity is produced by means of epidemic controls such as social distancing and fluctuating mandates about permissible gathering sizes, quarantine rules, and mask-wearing dictates. It is not an exaggeration to speak of the covidisation of subjectivation by means of public health models converted into means – the exercise of public health powers; use of regulations; setting fines, threats, and inducements; managing resistances of all sorts – of surveilling and controlling their citizenry by governments. New modes of collective subjectivation are being created in the midst of Covid such as safe cohorts, social bubbles, but also a new type of 'machinic solitude' (Guattari 1996: 267) in the proliferations of web seminars, virtual meetings, and so on that inflect the already advanced 'mutation of subjectivity' brought about according to Guattari by computerisation, but evident today in the robots that sanitise public places, detect the absence of masks, or dispense health information. So-called machinic isolation entails in many cases varying durations of quarantine and self-isolation combined with greater use of social media and remote shopping, the latter in some ways exacerbating the spread of the virus through poor working conditions in fulfilment centres.

What Is Metamodelling?

Schizoanalysis is Guattarian metamodelling. Metamodelling is a critical approach to method that prioritizes the construction of diagrams in automodelisations, that is, self-engendering cartographies of subjectivation, with neither hard pre-existent nor final determinations, but with analytic relevance to processes of singularisation. Auto-modeling non-conforms to standard types. Auto-modeling is not, and Guattari insists on this point, 'an alternative modelization' (Guattari 1996: 133). It is not just another model with a program to which it begs or buys allegiance.

Guattari writes: 'schizoanalysis only poses one question: how does one model oneself?' (1996: 132). Myth-derived models from psychoanalysis explain how one may be tethered to familial constructs. Large and small models of membership, from nation to neighbourhood, inform a sense of belonging. Such references are myths, narratives, identities, roles. These can be imaginary. They can arise and erode at any time. They are loved and hated, sought after and avoided. As a metamodel schizoanalysis, Guattari writes:

> tries to understand how it is that you got where you are? "What is your model to you?" It does not work? – Then, I don't know, one tries to work together. One must see if one can make a graft of other models. It will be perhaps better, perhaps worse. We will see. There is no question of posing a standard model. And the criterion of truth in this comes precisely when the meta-modelization transforms itself into auto-modelization, or auto-gestation, if you prefer.
>
> *(Guattari 1996: 133)*

He is neither concerned with inherited standards nor with new standards but considers grafting as an option, only as a step towards a kind of singular auto-modelling.

Guattari's discussion of models, especially in *Schizoanalytic Cartographies* (2013), is brief. It arises, however, in the context of the difference between schizoanalysis and various psychoanalytic schools. Schizoanalysis is not another specialism or school of thought certifying technicians; Guattari does not want to find a place, a 'rank' for it in the 'psy domain' (Guattari 2013: 17).

In detaching schizoanalysis from an 'institutional foundation', Guattari exposes its critical mission: 'to become a discipline for reading other modelling systems … an instrument for deciphering modelling systems in diverse domains' (2013: 17). Guattari is not offering a philosophy of modelling. It is more like a critical comparative approach to reading models, but his goal is to direct metamodelling toward encouraging and understanding self-organization.

Erin Manning (2016: 67) inserts Guattari's conception of metamodelling into her analysis of the limits of method in the first chapter of her book, *The Minor Gesture*. 'Schizoanalysis was Guattari's antimodel position', she writes, a 'proposition that would upset existing formations of power and knowledge'. Guattari's understanding of the strong gravitational pull of models arose within the context of a combination of theory-building and clinical practice, as normative and predetermined obstacles that required refutation. Shifting from antimodel to anti-method, Manning (2016: 67) specifies that 'metamodeling is against method, active in its refutation of pre-existing modes of existence'. Guattari sometimes suggested that metamodel and anti-method could be used interchangeably, especially in his more free-wheeling discussions, some of which Manning quotes from his interview with Jacques Pain; however, the two terms are not interchangeable. Metamodelling can give rise, according to Guattari (1996: 122), to an 'analytic methodology' that is built upon the inflection of metamodelling as a critical practice that refutes the representational logic of existing models. Metamodelling works against the grain of the pre-existent in order to attend to felt passages, variations over rules, beyond the edges of meaning and disciplinarity. An 'analytic methodology' is not an anti-method as such; rather, it is 'more of a procedure of auto-modelization which appropriates all or part of existing models in order to construct its own cartographies, its own reference points, and thus its own analytic approach' (Guattari 1996: 122). Metamodelling grafts bits of or even entire models onto other models. Grafting is a process of alignment that generates hybridization. We can take Manning's claim another way: metamodelling is neither a general method nor an anti-method. The question of method is not an easy one to answer. Franco Berardi (2008: 114), for instance, refers to schizoanalysis as a 'psychotherapeutic method, but also a way of conceiving of the relationship between singularity and its chaosmosis, that is, its conceptual, artistic, psychic, existential, political, relational and linguistic creations. …' The singularity of psychogenesis requires a singular method, one that renders fluid solid models: 'If chaosmosis is the process through which singular creativity gives its own order to the chaotic constellations that circumscribe the conscious organism, then schizoanalysis proposes to act as an ecology of the mind and a therapy of becoming world' (Berardi 2008: 114). This notion of therapy does not, it is worth emphasizing, pursue an ideal of scientificity from which schizoanalysis is to be protected. Rather, it is aesthetic, poetic to be precise in Berardi's hands, and magical in Guattari's (2013: 32) hands, which functioned for him as an antidote to standards of psychotherapeutic scientific professionalism. The question for him was where one goes after ridding oneself of 'every scientific reference' when mapping subjectivity. For Guattari, that would be animism, magic, and hypnosis.

Schizoanalysis attempts to diagram the process of subjectivation by looking critically at assemblages of enunciation, inter-assemblage relationships, and how they impact context-embedded semiotic productions. Guattari calls this 'metamodelling trans-assemblage relations' (2013: 20). Subjectivation here is used in the Guattarian sense of an assemblage of diverse components, noting that many will not have 'consciousness' or other traditional attributes of a thinking subject: 'the assemblage of enunciation will thus be led to 'exceed' the problematic of the individuated subject' (2013: 18). Thinking and enunciation may be displaced onto informational phyla, in platform algorithms and machinic orality, for instance. Guattari (2013: 40) calls this signaletic matter, which he contrasts with optional matter, the 'logics of self-reference' that can neither be represented nor indexed to outside referents (discursivised).

The Covidisation of Subjectivation

How would Guattari decipher subjectivation in the time of Covid? The semiotic remodelling of sociality takes place directly though governmental incursions into existential territories by means of restricted travel, social distancing, quarantine, lockdowns, the entry of death into everyday spaces, and the troubling of the skinscape of handshakes, socio-sexual relations, and shared ventilation systems. Publicly available epidemic models provide semiotic support for these initiatives in the name of managing infection rates in relation to hospital capacity and the master signifier of the R – basic reproduction number – despite its inferential imprecision (i.e., extent of infection, but not its speed). But it remains a politically potent whip nonetheless to which public policy may be lashed and restrictions on the population tightened or loosened as the number fluctuates around a factor of 1 (Adam 2020). The mental health fallout has been slow to emerge but is clearly a major factor shaping future social relations. Schizoanalytic metamodelling would look closely at the pragmatics of submission to models entailing restrictions during Covid in order to understand the effects on assemblages of enunciation and look for resources available for exploratory semiotisations.

I have already mentioned disturbances to inter-assemblage relations under curtailed conditions of stay-at-home messages (the meaning of 'home' is never really properly parsed), but it is worth considering the ways in which potentialities around metabolic encounters are truncated yet at the same time deflected into forms of remote contact by digital means while working from home or by mediations of layered personal protective equipment, and the small measure of creativity some of these afford. Information machines are shaping existential territories by bringing into central circulation the role of video conferencing platforms where they would otherwise remain peripheral. Personal health information is now more exposed than ever to police surveillance and corporate misuse; new forms of surveillance blossom like wastewater detection, previously used extensively for drug detection, to the Covid virus, redefining neighbourhoods, blocks, buildings, and residences as 'hotspots' but without any social or political analysis. While biomedical models assist in the deterritorialisation of encounters when they are crudely politically translated, resistant subjectivations also arise. Union organizing is advancing during Covid as many unrepresented frontline workers see that workplace safety is a key issue, not to mention their suppressed wages and poor benefits (Guattari's remarks on union experiments are notable; 1996: 270). A renewed interest in the refusal of work has emerged, despite difficulties in its enforcement, even in jurisdictions that permit it due to health concerns.

The Black Lives Matter collective has emerged as a broker of what Guattari (1996: 272) called 'ecosophic democracy' by advancing 'dissensual metamodelizations' in the form of multiple campaigns such as Defund the Police and Breathe Day. BLM has in some respects liberated the unconscious by bringing it into contact with the realities of structural racism and calling forth the need for solidarity in the struggle for the revalorisation of Black experience in the face of overt and covert violence. And Scholar Strike in the US and Canada was one answer to this call back in September 2020 and 2022. #Say Their Names and Say Her Name, and related enunciative protests against anti-Black racism, are refrains that are designed to trigger refusals of the white patriarchical status quo. Guattari's interest in the existential dimensions of orality may be appreciated in saying the names of Black victims of state violence which fills back in and re-energizes the semiotic polyvocality of their lives, protecting them from overcoding by hostile agents (Guattari 1995: 89). From reviving a civil rights gesture of taking a knee to saying their names, resistant semiotic components have been regained and released not only for the sake of the struggle against racism but in the service of overcoming in general reactionary impulses and expanding narrow points of view.

Ecosophy in the Covid-19 Era

Metamodelling in the time of Covid necessitates a shift into syndemic thinking of the relationships between biological and social factors impacting public health. As Richard Horton (2020: 874) wrote in *The Lancet*:

> The most important consequence of seeing Covid-19 as a syndemic is to underline its social origins. The vulnerability of older citizens; Black,

> Asian, and minority ethnic communities; and key workers who are commonly poorly paid with fewer welfare protections points to a truth so far barely acknowledged – namely, that no matter how effective a treatment or protective a vaccine, the pursuit of a purely biomedical solution to Covid-19 will fail.

This opens the reading or deciphering of epidemic models to the forces of resistant sujbectivations exposing racial and socioeconomic inequalities and ongoing state violence that support standardised capitalist subjectivities. If by deciphering we can also understand debunking the supposed non-prejudicial nature of the virus: Covid actually discriminates through a disproportionate infection rate among the most vulnerable groups, when sheltering in place heightens susceptibility; when existing health inequities due to racism imperil Black lives.

Considering the pandemic as a syndemic requires an opening to ecosophical thinking. Guattari's (2000: 42) three 'interchangeable lenses' of ecosophy, mental, and social and environmental ecologies, might suggest, under the threat of Covid, a 'unifying objective' such as the development of vaccines and how they are rolled out and distributed (2000: 34). Guattari warned against reducing solutions to the application of greater and greater techno-scientific power. He was also wary of blind faith in pharmaceutical companies, as well as in the state administrators who control the distribution of vaccines. At present, the lessons from police and state violence against protesters, rationalised on the basis of the protection of critical infrastructure, are returning to organise vaccine access around a contested blend of the susceptibility of employment groups to the virus, security concerns, and characterisations of the lack of symbolic worth of certain populations (i.e., working poor, prisoners).

At the same time, he did not recoil from contemporary conditions in which technology, science, labour, nature, and culture have changed fundamentally and rapidly over the past few decades. Guattari referred to environmental ecology, for instance, not in terms one might expect, borrowed from nature loving, conservation, or even political or media ecologies, but as machinic ecology, a complex entanglement of human and natural (cosmic) relationships on a planetary scale. In order to intervene in times of crisis, Guattari (2000: 66) warned that 'vast programmes will need to be set up in order to regulate the relationship between oxygen, ozone and carbon dioxide in the Earth's atmosphere'. While such quasi-global accords have been achieved, such as the 2016 Paris Agreement on climate change, this has not stopped major greenhouse gas emitting countries from threatening to pull out, or from accelerating rainforest destruction in the name of short-term political agendas, such as the Bolsonaro government in Brazil between 2019 and 2023. Throughout the pandemic, the World Health Organization has played an important informational and organizational role. Its COVAX Advance Market Commitment supports many small and medium national economies to ensure vaccine procurement, but it is far from global (indeed, the skewed distribution rehearses the divide between a handful of wealthy countries and the remainder of the world, only a few of the latter managing well with non-pharmaceutical means). Still, this is the kind of initiative that Guattari anticipated would be required to address large-scale challenges, especially under the distorting influence of intrusive capitalistic goals, neo-conservatisms of the sort that the Trump administration introduced in the United States. If 2020 marked 40 years of research into HIV/AIDS without a vaccine, despite all of the weight of UNAIDS, WHO, conferences, declarations, funds, self-tests, treatment regimes, and unmet targets, Guattari's statements about the urgency of the fight against AIDS in the 1980s are still relevant now, at the very moment when the altruistic prospect of sharing vaccines seems so fraught.

Metamodelisation scouts out points of rupture in dominant significations that can radically remake how a rapidly covidised subjectivity can auto-model itself. The outline of this micropolitical perspective presented here is projective, pointing to a Guattarian way of understanding and responding to the syndemic. This is not a call to break quarantine or abandon masks. On the contrary, it is a strategy of deciphering and breaking through imposed significations and rearranging their components, how one contends with the uncertainties of an ongoing situation and its overt territorial reinscriptions; singular cartographies can be drawn in the encounter with adversity, including the potential for social change, keeping in mind Guattari's recognition of the difficulties of holding these together in a novel situation where questions of social cohesion are unavoidable (Guattari 1995: 132).

The social includes, however, inter-species relationships. If Covid-19 has its dynamic points of origin in so-called wet markets – open air markets where animals are traded live and/or butchered for sale, some of which trade in (legal and illegal) wildlife and mix these animals with domesticates raised for food – inter-species contagion is a key factor in Covid subjectivation. It is not a question of eliminating these markets. Not only are these local food systems which exist outside of the industrial food complex critical for the under-served populations that rely on them, but attention to zoonotic leaps of viruses in them opens up a vast field of emerging, not yet established, diseases, which makes coronavirus the tip of a pathogenic iceberg and calls for the recentering of non-human–human species relations on the international agenda, engaging wildlife law, animal welfare, and food security and pointing the way to widespread production and growing availability of cultured meats.

Guattari (2000: 62) issued an ecosophical caution about the 'machinization of time' that would influence the emergence of new subjectivities. His brief observations rest on the emergence of the role of time in immaterial labour, as well as on the temporalities of control societies – the shift from disciplinary temporal ordering (timetables) to cyberneticised temporal regimes that engage digital technologies which extend, modify, and inflect microphysics of power into mobile modulatory forms. This general process of dematerialisation, unbinding, and flexibilisation of time takes place through the myriad applications of coded information, from platforms to passwords. But Covid is also part of this regime. On the level of temporality, it is a novel viral time, as Michael J. Flexer (2020: 4) has trenchantly described it:

> Viral time is not a metaphoric association between the viral action within our cells and the impact of a pandemic on our lives; it is the literal infection, proliferation and enforcement of the temporality of the virus on our social conventions.

During Covid, a syndemic that arrived before it arrived, time has become unstable, it is counted differently, through daily infection and death rates, through holiday cancellations, and the broader crises of the social, labour, and capitalist production, not to mention the crisis of imagining post-pandemic futures. Indeed, regimes of time linked to modelled projections, isolation timelines, quarantine reporting periods, symptom timelines, are imposed on viral time to flatten, to plank, to crush it. Flexer wants to imagine viral time's potential for revolution, for making history, insofar as

> time has come to a standstill and can now take a stand. Being liberated from a future means also being liberated from the past. Revolutions … change from impossible to inevitable in one beat less than a heartbeat; they have already arrived as the only living time.
>
> *(2020: 8)*

Turning back to Guattari, let's consider this break as a coupure (cut or break) by shrinking ourselves to molecular revolutionary size, away from the capital R revolution of Lenin, Bolsheviks, and October, and regain this moment of reversal from viral to living time. But this is to understand break in terms of a signifying cut, which can be only discovered by following what happens to the signifier. Something happens to the signifier, then, in viral time, that separates a potentially revolutionary breakthrough from evolutionary, developmental history, the latter on the side of the signified and repetition, and the former on that of changes in meaning and socio-semiotic pragmatics. 'But that signifying break is as hard to identify as the underlying meaning of a dream', admits Guattari (2015: 241). He goes to some length to show how uncertain the situation had been with the regard to the weakness of the Russian bourgeoisie for Lenin, his actions against his own party, and so on. So, then, what are the 'carriers' of such breakthroughs? This Guattarian signifier is not reducible to structural linguistics; rather, it is a 'raw material' that can be 'remolded' into many other substances, and only the ramifications of this breach can really affect the signified. It is hardly a signifier at all, but more of a diagram with iconic and indexical properties. This remade signifier does not lose its structural affiliation with subjectivation as Guattari retains this feature of Lacanian thought. Thus, time must have some impact on subjectivation. Guattari's sense of cut is an interruption in 'historical causality' but punctuated by temporal markers: the 'ten days that shook the world', and 'the hour of the first socialist revolution', and so on.

Studies of time perception during Covid suggest that distortions (slowing linked to increased age, decreased task load, negative affect around diminishing socialization, increased stress, increased task load that would normally speed up time's passage, and stress may interact counter-intuitively) are widely experienced (Ogden 2020). These psychosocial studies do not reach into Guattari's understanding of subjectivation as fundamentally de-centered from the human. This is marked by his deployment of the term *machinic*: 'it is not essentially centered on human subjectivity, and it puts into play material fluxes and the most diverse social systems' (2009: 141). Temporal distortions and instabilities that reach beyond human perception open up experience to non-human animal and artifactual rhythms and passages. The machinic temporality of subjectivation during viral time cannot amount to either working class or revolutionary subjectivity in the traditional sense. Rather, the components of this kind of subjectivity (neither 'exceptional' nor 'homogeneous') include heterogeneous non-normal temporalities (Guattari 2011: 158–159). With the roll-out of a variety of vaccines, the two-step rhythm of vaccination, coupled with the spectre of annual boosters, diagrams a future unfurling of pandemic focused life, within the cellular process of building immunity.

Assemblages of temporalisation during Covid may be described in accordance with Guattari's threefold set of directions that their machinic nuclei tend towards:

i. Hyper-territorialised subjectivations: personalised involutions in which time perception slows down and even stops in restricted spaces (quarantine sleep disturbances);
ii. Chronographic enslavement: enslaved by capitalistic refrains set into motion through the move to online, extension of screen time and its syndromes (Zoom fatigue), to the extent of becoming a component part of machinic relays (surveillance) and exchanges (online ordering and delivery networks);
iii. Rhizomatic mutations: imagining new relationships to capitalist refrains by weakening the magnification of inequalities through small data gathering about challenges faced by excluded marginalized populations, perhaps in the spirit of an ACT UP Covid for sexual and gender minorities;

heightened use of refusal to work and protected leave policies in the face of unsafe working conditions, leading to novel molecular connections through all of the ways of desiring creation.

Conclusion: Unglued Alterities and Deterritorialised Assemblages

Metamodelling tells us that there can be no general model circulated that would further opportunities for auto-modelling during Covid. Indeed, for Guattari (2016: 102), 'the idea of a "model" for self-management is thus contradictory'. It would be contradictory for a meta-modeller to invoke a tree model for self-management. Further, metamodelling is not yet another model, say a rhizome, as it is a graft of another model or part of it onto an existing model, a rhizome–tree hybrid. Guattari is not searching for replacement models. Metamodelling the pandemic requires grafts, but a question remains: Which models accommodate grafts better than others? What happens when grafts don't take? Even the most standard of models can accept grafts, such as the SIR model of Covid spread (susceptible–infected–recovered, each group with different rates of change), but also an exposed group, which introduces a new equation in-between susceptible and infected. Grafting onto a failing model, one whose assumptions are wrong and produce exaggerations, like homogenous infection among the population, thus fails many people at risk. Writing in *The New England Journal of Medicine*, Inga Holmdahl and Caroline Buckee (2020) invoke a classic modelling nomenclature – 'wrong but useful' – to tackle where things went awry: poor knowledge of the virus' behaviour and location of uncertainty in the model (i.e., immunity periods, asymptomatic infection rates, contacts between susceptible and infected). For a metamodeller, questioning expertise is an obvious first step, not to foment paranoid reactive protests but to expose the (mis)fit between modelling and policy, that is, between epidemiology and policy (i.e., the use of lockdowns), that could be taken advantage of by authoritarian populists who wanted to increase police powers or give advantages to their supporters. Unlike the scientific and social scientific communities, however, a Guattarian metamodeller will push modelling so far that it evolves into 'a new map for each analysis', as Janell Watson explains (2013: 191), connecting them with social forces, machines, and arts in generating many analytic cartographies of Covid subjectivations.

The series of lockdowns, curfews, and other restrictions that continue to impinge on territorial assemblages are forces of deterritorialisation that impact social relations. Scaled back into a circumscribed existential territory (familiar like a home or apartment, or even unfamiliar in a forced quarantine shelter such as a hotel), new existential refrains are encountered in the mixed temporalities previously mentioned, the new faces of masked family, friends, neighbours, and strangers, as well as the health experts and leaders so prevalent in the media, not to mention the gridded faces or black boxes of video conferencing platforms. The Covidised subject is a terminal through which these heterogeneous temporalities and faces flow and beat, given the limited physical alterities available, the collapsed refrains of domestic territories, and the impingements of capitalistic refrains of e-commerce that overcode holiday celebrations. Assailed by machinic faciality traits in the form of masks that become redundant refrains, Covidised subjects either elect to join, or to dispute, this trans-subjective, de-individuating, yet social assemblage as a way to regain some measure of a-syndemic time and space, for better and for worse. Collective experimentation and exploration, across sectors and social movements, for instance, through online health hackathons (#WirVsVirus), without getting mired in disavowals of the entrepreneurial state, and corporate acceleration of artificial intelligence driven agendas, can further critiques of neo-liberalism and return to normality narratives.

References

Adam, David. 2020. 'A guide to R, the pandemic's misunderstood metric'. *Nature* (03 July): 1–14. https://www.nature.com/articles/d41586-020-02009-w. Accessed December 22, 2020.

Berardi, Franco. 2008. *Félix Guattari: Thought, Friendship and Visionary Cartography*. Translated by G. Mecchia and C. J. Stivale. London: Palgrave Macmillan.

Flexer, Michael J. 2020, June 10. 'Having a moment: The revolutionary semiotic of COVID-19'. *Wellcome Open Research*, 5: 134. https://doi.org/10.12688/wellcome openres.15972.1. Accessed on December 9, 2020.

Guattari, Félix. 1995. *Chaosmosis*. Translated by P. Bains and J. Pefanis. Bloomington: Indiana University Press.

Guattari, Félix. 1996. *The Guattari Reader*. Gary Genosko (eds.). Oxford: Blackwell.

Guattari, Félix. 2000. *The Three Ecologies*. Translated by I. Pindar and P. Sutton. London: Athlone.

Guattari, Félix. 2009. *Les Années d'Hiver 1980–85*. Paris: Les Prairies Ordinaires.

Guattari, Félix. 2011. *The Machinic Unconscious*. Translated by T. Adkins. Los Angeles: Semiotext(e).

Guattari, Félix. 2013. *Schizoanalytic Cartographies*. Translated by A. Goffey. London: Bloomsbury.

Guattari, Félix. 2015. *Psychoanalysis and Transversality*. Translated by Ames Hodges. Los Angeles: Semiotext(e).

Guattari, Félix. 2016. *Lines of Flight: For Another World of Possibilities*. Translated by A. Goffey, London: Bloomsbury.

Holmdahl, Inga and Caroline Buckee. 2020. 'Wrong but Useful: What Covid-19 Epidemiologic Models Can and Cannot Tells Us'. *The New England Journal of Medicine* 383: 3030–3035.

Manning, Erin. 2016. *The Minor Gesture*. Durham: Duke University Press.

Morgan, Mary S. 2012. *The World in the Model: How Economists Work and Think*. New York: Cambridge University Press.

Ogden, Ruth S. 2020. 'The Passage of Time During the UK Covid-19 Lockdown'. *PLOS ONE* 15/7: 1–16.

Richard Horton, Richard. 2020, September 26. 'Offline: COVID-19 Is Not a Pandemic'. *The Lancet* 396/10255: 874. https://www.thelancet.com/journals/lancet/article/PIIS0140-6736(20)32000-6/fulltext. Accessed December 22, 2020.

Watson, Janell. 2013. 'Metamodelization' in Eugene B. Young, Gary Genosko and Janell Watson (eds.), *The Deleuze & Guattari Dictionary*, 191–192. London: Bloomsbury.

4

THE COVID-19 PANDEMIC AND MEDICO-CYBER-POLITICAL DISCOURSE

Kenneth Surin

The Covid-19 pandemic has introduced new and complicated theoretical and practical spaces in which medical sciences (such as virology) combine with a new kind of 'algorithmic reason' (deployed, e.g., in track-and-trace apps) and political practices and discourses to constitute a novel medico-cyber-political assemblage combining practical and discursive elements.[1]

This assemblage has breached somewhat established demarcations between medical science, the pharmaceutical industry, computerised communicative networks, and politics. For one thing, it is clear that the medical sciences involved, which were politicised from the outset, were always in the realm of a political (as opposed to a purely medical) discourse. For another, the epidemiology of Covid-19 relies heavily on computerised algorithms for its track-and-trace apps, though again the use and control of these apps were heavily inserted into political decision-making. In the UK, for instance, much has been made of the creation of (botched) track-and-trace apps, as well as other dismal failures, all entrusted to unqualified cronies and donors of the ruling Tory party – to mention a single example, the landlord of the local pub of the health minister, Matt Hancock, had a contract to supply PPE thrown into his lap by his prominent customer, the aforementioned health minister. Discourses regarding Covid-19 are thus inextricably medico-cyber-political discourses of a hybrid nature, straddling and combining many areas of medicine, myriad computerised systems, applications, and a messy and often corrupt politics. I'll draw on Deleuze and Guattari's use of Louis Hjelmslev's semiotics to map out and analyse this new discursive terrain. But first, by way of some initial footwork, the question of producing a concept needs to be broached.[2] Deleuze and Guattari are explicit about relating the genesis of a

DOI: 10.4324/9781003507789-5

concept to the *event* of its production. To quote at some length a relevant passage from their *What Is Philosophy?*:

> The philosopher is the concept's friend; he is the potentiality of the concept. That is, philosophy is not the simple art of forming, inventing, or fabricating concepts, because concepts are not necessarily forms, discoveries, or products. More rigorously, philosophy is the discipline that involves *creating* concepts. ... The object of philosophy is to create concepts that are always new. ... Concepts are not waiting for us ready-made, like heavenly bodies. There is no heaven for concepts. They must be invented, fabricated, or rather created. ... Nietzsche laid down the task of philosophy when he wrote, "[Philosophers] must no longer accept concepts as a gift, nor merely purify and polish them, but first *make* and *create* them, present them and make them convincing. Hitherto one has generally trusted one's concepts as if they were a wonderful dowry from some sort of wonderland," but trust must be replaced by distrust, and philosophers must distrust most those concepts they did not create themselves.
>
> *(Deleuze and Guattari 1994: 5–6*[3]*)*

If we proceed in accordance with this Deleuzo-Guattarian prescription, we will need to distinguish adequately between (1) the concepts of a *theory* of X (X could be a medical science, or a national cinema or whatever), (2) the concepts *intrinsic* to X (i.e., a particular medical science such as virology or a specific national cinema, etc.) and (3) that particular medical science or national cinema in its barest and most irreducible empirical or material *conditions*.

A theory of X is something that is produced or created no less than its putative object X. It is a practice, just as a medical science (e.g., virology) is a multilinear ensemble of practices. A theory, to be more precise, is a practice of concepts. A theory of a medical science is not "about" that medical science, but about the *concepts* that medical science happens to generate, concepts that are themselves related in more or less complex ways to other practices and so on. A theory, in short, operates on the concepts integral to the practical expression of this or that medical science.

A *theory* of virology does not therefore impinge directly on the sheerly empirical phenomena constituting virology, but on the concepts generated by the virological field, which, however, are no less practical, actual, or effective than virology itself. (This is simply another way of registering in a way that is as unavoidable as it is problematic that scarcely deniable affectivity of 'thought' with which the 'idealist' philosophical traditions have always been impressed, but which their materialist counterparts have found embarrassing or not susceptible to adequate description and analysis, or else reducible in principle to something more fundamental and compelling, namely, 'matter'.)

Virology's concepts are not given in the assemblages of practices that constitute it, yet they are virology's concepts, not theories about virology. Every medical science generates for itself its own 'thinkability' (and concomitantly its own 'unthinkability' as the obverse of this very 'thinkability'), and its concepts are constitutive of that 'thinkability'. Another way of making this point would be to say that a medical science has to secrete its myriad expressivities precisely in order to be able to be what it is and that its concepts—in ways that are inevitably selective, limiting, and even arbitrary—are the thematizations or representations of these expressivities. Or, more generally, the concepts of a medical science are its expressivities rendered in the form of that science's 'thinkability'.

Theories of virology, by contrast, are *theories* produced by reflection on the natures, functions, and so forth of these expressivities. They operate on a particular medical science's 'thinkability'. It is fine and salutary to ask the question 'What is virology?' but there is another kind of question to be asked as well, in this case 'What is (a) theory of (virology)?' Virology itself is an immensely varied and complex practice of signs whose theory philosophers of science and historians of medicine and others must produce, but produce precisely as conceptual practice. No theoretical determination, no matter how subtle or thorough, can on its own constitute the concepts of virology.[4] As indicated, these concepts are expressed in advance and independently of theoretical practice. Theorists, qua theorists, can only traffic in theories of medicine (or religion or cinema).

The concepts that theorists deal with can function in more than one field of thought, and even in a single domain it is always possible for a concept to fulfill more than one function. For example, depending on the context, the concept 'virus' can function in fields as diverse as virology (of course), but also epidemiology, forensic criminology, public health and safety, computer science, various technologies of imaging, and so on. Each variable of thought is of course defined by its own internal variables, variables that have a complex relation to their external counterparts (such as clinical infrastructures, university laboratories, political and social conditions and forces, even the sheer physical state of things). (It is tempting here to understand this complexity in terms that are akin to Althusser's sense of the 'overdetermined' relation between formations.) It follows that a concept comes into being or ceases to be effective only when there is a change of function and/or field. Functions for concepts must be created or abolished for them to be generated or eliminated, and new fields must be brought into being in order for concepts to be rendered irrelevant or invalid.

All the foregoing seems like a long-drawn-out clearing of the throat, but I'm not saying anything really new here—Foucault's *Les mots et les choses* contains a now famous depiction of visibility that conforms in outline to my somewhat perfunctory accounts of function and field. There Foucault discredits the age-old conception of visibility as something that has its origins in a general/generative source of light that casts itself upon and thereby 'illuminates' pre-existing objects. For Foucault, visibility is determined by an apparatus (*dispositif*) that has its own particular way of structuring light, determining the way in which it falls, spreads, and obscures; an apparatus that demarcates the visible from the invisible, in this way bringing into being entire arrays of objects with this or that mode of visibility as their condition of possibility; a scopic apparatus or regime that also causes objects to be wholly or partially effaced, hidden. Hence even something so taken for granted and innocuous as the very visibility of things is created by an apparatus or regime, in this case a scopic regime, which provides 'rules' that govern the very existence and operating conditions of visibility. (And these conditions, as Foucault himself never tired of pointing out, are always 'political'.) It seems obvious that the notion of the *concept* itself likewise conforms to such 'rules' for the generation and perpetuation of concepts.[5]

Deleuze attributes to Louis Hjelmslev an insightful modification of Saussure's account of the linguistic sign, by taking the novel and significant step of incorporating nonlinguistically formed matter or sense ('purport') into the study of semiosis. From *Logique du sens* to *Anti-Oedipus* (his collaboration with Guattari), Deleuze sought a theory of an a-signifying, 'pure designation' falling within the poststructuralist remit. Hjelmslev in his *Prolegomena to a Theory of Language* used the term 'purport' to refer to both the unstructured phonic stuff or mass of the plane of expression and the amorphous 'thought-mass' (Saussure's *pensée*) of the plane of content. Hjelmslev, says Deleuze, therefore developed an account of semiosis capable of delineating the deictic or indexical (the use of words and phrases to refer to a specific time, place, or person in context, e.g., the words *tomorrow*, *there*, or *they*); the connotative (the feeling evoked by a word or phrase); and the demonstrative or denotative (words or phrases that point to a specific object); as functions of signs – as well as their *autonomy* with regard to the powers of signification (i.e., the representation of this or that meaning) possessed by the signs in question.

The functions of signs:

- The deictic or indexical – the use of words and phrases to refer to a specific time, place, or person in context; 3xamples: the words *tomorrow*, *there*, or *they*
- The connotative – the feeling evoked by a word or phrase
- The demonstrative or denotative – words or phrases that point to a specific object
- All signs – the indexical, the connotative, the denotative – possess an autonomy regarding the powers of signification (i.e., the representation of this or that meaning) possessed by the signs in question

HJELMSLEV: THE LINGUISTIC SYSTEM

'HOSPITAL'

EXPRESSION	→	content – 'Pathologies'
(sayability)	→	form/signified – 'Medicine'
CONTENT	→	form/signifier – 'Clinic', 'hospital'
(visibility)	→	content – Patients

HJELMSLEV: THE LINGUISTIC SYSTEM (A MESS WHEN IT COMES TO COVID-19?)

'COVID-19'

EXPRESSION	→	content – 'Pathology' (evidence-based science, hoax/ fake, big pharma scam, etc.)
(sayability)	→	form/signified – 'Medicines' (several vaccines, Regeneron, steroids, experimental treatments still underway)
CONTENT	→	form/signifier – 'Clinic', 'hospital' (National University Hospital Singapore/ Mayo Clinic)
(visibility)	→	content – Patients (but which ones?)

This all seems like a bit of a mess, but Hjelmslev's notion of 'purport' allows a way out. It will be recalled Hjelmslev used the term 'purport' to refer both to the unstructured phonic stuff or mass of the plane of expression and the amorphous 'thought-mass' (Saussure's *pensée*) of the plane of content. But first a rough-and-ready intellectual history, preceded by a short excursus on the Deleuzo-Guattarian account of the production of narrative-concepts.

The intellectual-historical conditions for the production of the (Deleuzean and Deleuzo-Guattarian) narrative-concept are to be found at the core of the preceding philosophical tradition. According to this tradition, the being of a particular, qua particular, can only be registered passively through human intuition – I can have a grasp of a particular only by having an actual experience of the particular in question. Concepts, however, can be employed independently of any actual experience and do not depend on the passive sensible receptivity of an empirical 'given' for their use – in Kant's words, concepts are marked by a productive 'spontaneity', in contrast to the non-creative 'passivity' of sensible intuitions.[6] Deleuze is certainly not the first philosopher who sought to dismantle this dichotomy between concept and intuition, and it is now something of a commonplace to say that Heidegger is the contemporary philosopher who more than any other elevated this dismantling into the quintessential philosophical 'project'. But Heidegger's basis for this dismantling is still placed within the confines of a phenomenological ontology, that is, he sought to answer the question 'how is receptivity possible?' by resorting to the notion of the pre-givenness of being, and in the process could not account for the productive processes that underlie sensibility itself. For Deleuze, by contrast, the central task of philosophy is precisely the creation of a metaphysics capable of accounting for these productive processes.

The problem with this separation between concept and intuition, or *noesis* and *aisthesis*, is one that has permeated the very core of the philosophical tradition. The age-old distinctions between epistemology and aesthetics, (true) judgment and (mere) taste, all have their basis in this separation. And just as venerable are the attempts to overcome this disconnection, an attempt nowhere more apparent than in Kant's realization that he needed to write a *Critique of Judgment* (to wit, aesthetic judgment) to 'complete' the project that began with his *Critique of Pure Reason* (dealing of course with judgment in the domain of truth governed by reason). For Deleuze, the attempts to overcome the dichotomy between (general) concept and (particular) sensible intuition are bound to fail, and this because the principles devised in this philosophical 'overcoming' succumb to unavoidable metaphysical illusions. The most common of these illusions involves the use of abstract concepts to group together isolated particulars. These abstract concepts – Being, Unity, Thought, Matter, and so forth – are then inevitably bestowed an a priori ontological superiority denied to the metaphysically inferior particulars, and this because notions like Being and Unity and so on are simply not 'given' in immediate experience, and thus must be positioned as a pure exteriority transcending the contents of immediate experience.[7] There is no way round or out of this predicament as long as the distinction between (transcendent) *noesis* and (transcended) *aisthesis* is retained, and Deleuze opts instead to cut the Gordian knot by assigning to the concept a totally different function and status.

Rather than giving the abstract concept the policing or custodial rôle accorded it by the previous philosophical tradition, Deleuze prefers to abandon the tradition's static view of the concept as purely designative, or denominative, or descriptive, and instead views the concept as active and creative. A concept for Deleuze (and Guattari) has three intertwined components: a 'possible world, existing face, and real language or speech' (Deleuze and Guattari 1994: 20). A field of experience on their view is always related to a simple 'there is'. Hence, if I experience fear now that the Covid-19 virus has reached the place where I live (Blacksburg, Virginia), then it is a condition of having this experience that there is such a thing as the Covid virus, that there is a place (Blacksburg) which happens to be my place of residence, and so forth. But this world, the world that *is*, is always in a position to be interrupted and transformed – someone who gazes at it with a look of fear opens up the possibility of a frightening world, a look of fascination at the virus's capacity to spread in a rapid and seemingly arbitrary fashion opens up the possibility of a fascinating world, a look of grief at the loss of a loved one opens up the possibility of a grieving world, and so on. Thus, the frightening world in which the Covid virus comes to Blacksburg can be transformed into a world of hope when I find out that there is an ample supply of the Pfizer vaccine my local hospital, that the known cases of Covid in Blacksburg and the surrounding towns have been quarantined in effective ways, and so on, so that I now gaze on the (Covid) world (of Blacksburg) with a look of hope. Likewise, India is a possible world (it also happens of course to be a constituent of the actual world), one that becomes real when Hindu or Urdu or Tamil are spoken or India is mentioned within a given realm of experience (a high-school geography lesson, viewing a Bollywood film, etc.). A possible world is expressed by a face that gazes on a situation (with a look of fear, or fascination, hope, or grief, or whatever), and it takes shape in a language that makes it real (in the way that 'India' is made real by those who speak an Indian language or when it is spoken about in a given domain of experience).

A concept also has a relationship to other concepts by virtue of the shared problems addressed by the concepts in question – hence the concepts 'Covid virus' and 'public health' are related to each other in a 'problematics' constituted by the need to contain the virus by public health measures, but they have no such connection in a domain of experience where a hedge fund CEO says 'I am really hungry' as he opens the door to a Michelin three-star restaurant in London where the cheapest entrée costs seventy pounds (in this latter situation there would be a completely different 'problematic', namely, 'I am feeling hungry, but I'm looking forward to a splendid feast prepared by a celebrity chef', as opposed to the speech-forms inherent in a different 'problematics', whose typical mode of expression could be 'I am starving, but there's not even a bowl of soup to be had'). Concepts also relate to each other by having similar components:

> Concepts, which have only consistency or intensive ordinates outside of any coordinates, freely enter into relationships of nondiscursive resonance – either because the components of one become components with other heterogeneous components or because there is no difference of scale between them at any level. Concepts are centers of vibrations, each in itself and everyone in relation to all the others. This is why they all resonate rather than cohere or correspond with each other.
>
> *(Deleuze and Guattari 1994: 23[8])*

For example, the concepts 'being a sumo wrestler' and 'being an elephant' could have the element or component 'being massive' in common, though of course 'being a sumo wrestler' and 'being an elephant' may have little else in common (since as far as we know, elephants don't wrestle and sumo wrestlers don't have a trunk that can function as a water spout, etc.). There is thus no logically ordained relation between concepts. Hence, while 'This is a square circle' expresses a contradiction, this particular contradiction is manifested only when 'square' and 'circle' come to be related to each other in the same proposition, whereas the proposition 'In Kandinsky's painting *Bright Lucidity* a square is painted next to a circle' is certainly not contradictory. There is nothing intrinsic to 'square' and 'circle', as concepts, which requires them to resonate, or which prevents them from resonating, with each other, as they do in the case of Kandinsky's *Bright Lucidity*. For this reason, Deleuze insists that relationships between concepts are constitutively 'agrammatical'.

Since the 1960s tremendous strides have been made in the area of logic known as fuzzy logic, and its cognate area fuzzy semiotics – both the logic and the semiotics provide resources for theorizing the unstructured phonic stuff on Hjelmslev's plane of expression and the amorphous 'thought-mass' on his plane of content. Pioneering work in this area was done by Lotfi A. Zadeh (1921–2017), an Azerbaijani-born computer scientist, AI researcher, electrical engineer, logician, and mathematician who spent most of his academic career at Berkeley. Zadeh is widely regarded as the pioneer of the systematic study of imprecision and approximate or inexact reasoning, the problem of classifying objects in terms of categories that defy absolute precision, as well the question of imprecise boundaries between the categories in question (titled in classical bivalent logic as the challenge posed by 'imprecise predicates', which confounded this 'true or false' binary logic). Zadeh's work in computer science and AI led him to the insight that 'truth' has a value contingent upon the knowledge base within which it is positioned.[9]

The stepping-off point in a key area of fuzzy logic is the age-old sorites paradox:

* One grain of sand does not make a heap.
* If one grain doesn't make a heap, then two grains don't.
* If two grains don't make a heap, then three grains don't.

…

* If 999,999 grains don't make a heap, then 1 million grains don't.
* Therefore, 1 million grains don't make a heap.

The sorites paradox enables us to address the problematics of 'vagueness'.

To go back to our heap of sand example, what we see here is an inherent vagueness attaching to the concept of a heap of sand.

First, it is necessary to distinguish between 'vagueness' and 'ambivalence':

AMBIVALENCE – 'it could be A, but then it could also be B' (A and B are precise, but we don't which one is the case)

VAGUENESS – 'it is A, but potentially multiple values could be processed through A' (i.e., A is fundamentally imprecise)

All we've done here is insert a coda into Hjelmslev's schema to mark the constitutive imprecision that affects the schema when we apply it to the context provided by Covid-19.

Both ambivalence and vagueness are present in discourses about the Covid-19 pandemic. As an instance of the former, discussions about the virus's origins have involved at least two hypotheses: (1) animal-to-human transmission from an infected animal (object A) sold at the Wuhan fresh market; (2) a Covid-19 pathogen (object B) manufactured at the virological research institute in Wuhan that managed to infect a human being. Both the A and B in this scenario are precise in their constitution as objects, despite continued questions about their underlying aetiology. As an instance of the latter, the discovery of new strains of Covid-19 pose for investigators the question of which ones are more transmissible and virulent than others. For instance, there is growing evidence that the 'Indian variant' of the virus is spreading more quickly in London than the UK's own 'Kent variant'.[10] Laboratory investigators have thus to deal with data that may have an initial imprecision or vagueness before coming to more determinative conclusions. Another area of 'vagueness' in Covid vaccine production involved the time interval needed between administering the first and second doses of the vaccine in question (it should be noted that the Johnson & Johnson vaccine only involves a single dose) – how far could the second dose be delayed, so that more people could receive a first dose, in the hope that this will confer a degree of immunity on a larger section of the population? A further area of 'vagueness' involves the side-effects of the various vaccines, which of course can only be detected after a significant number of inoculations have been administered. A case in point here is a body of evidence suggesting that the AstraZeneca vaccine could be linked to the increased risk of blood clots. It may also be recalled how in the early stages of the pandemic researchers were looking into ways of understanding the differences between the Covid virus and the more virulent forms of common influenza, as a way of setting these apart from each other so that adequate prophylactics could be developed. At the same time researchers were investigating other recent mass virus outbreaks (e.g., Ebola and SARS) to ascertain if anything could be learned from the responses to Ebola and SARS. Historians of medicine and epidemiologists, using the latest methods of data-gathering, are also looking at previous pandemics, such as the devastating 1918 Spanish flu, to discover ostensible commonalities between that outbreak and today's Covid-19 pandemic.

A tool much used by epidemiologists tracking the transmission rates of the Covid-19 virus, vital for ascertaining the level of case-numbers that allow the 3 Ts (test–trace–track) to be managed, is the R 0 or basic reproduction number (BRN; of an infection, in this case the Covid-19 virus). This is the expected number of cases directly generated by a single case in a population where all individuals are susceptible to infection. For example, if a disease has an R 0 of 18, a person who has the disease will transmit it to an average of 18 other people. That replication will continue if no one has been vaccinated against the disease or is already immune to it in their community. There are three possibilities with regard to the R 0 number:

If R 0 is less than 1, each existing infection causes less than one new infection. In this case, the disease will decline and eventually die out. This referred to as 'flattening the curve' in layperson's terms.
If R 0 equals 1, each existing infection causes one new infection. The disease will stay alive and remain stable, but there won't be an outbreak or an epidemic, or an expansion of these. This too is called 'flattening the curve'.
If R 0 is more than 1, each existing infection causes more than one new infection. The disease will be transmitted between people, and there may be an outbreak or epidemic, or a growth of these.

It is obvious that an R 0 only delivers a number based on a data point that will more or less be out of date by the time the requisite calculations are finalized, given that infection rates are rarely static, and even if they are, it will take a future data point to arrive at the conclusion that an infection rate has remained the same. The BRN is always a snapshot of a point that has receded into the past. Another factor causing uncertainty in the rate of the trajectory of infection is the movement of undetected cases from a virus hotspot to other locations. In the US, college and university towns, many in rural areas, faced surges of Covid-19 cases when a significant proportion of their students returned from breaks in larger towns or cities, or during spring breaks at beach resorts that were hotspots for the virus. It will take a subsequent data point to produce an R 0 reflecting this latest situation.

A similar state of affairs exists in India, where the pandemic was out of control during its peak. A concern in India is the transmission of the virus to rural areas, as workers who migrated to the now highly infected cities in search of work flee these cities (having lost their jobs due to lockdowns) and return to their villages. Many of these workers will be returning to their villages with Covid-19 strains that are ravaging urban India, leading to record numbers of daily infections and the country's highest daily death tolls since the virus emerged.

India's rural areas are of course even more disadvantaged with regard to health and medical resources than its cities.

Moreover, deaths in rural areas, from whatever cause, are less likely to be registered than in bigger towns and cities, as more rural dwellers die at home without reaching a hospital, where the requisite bureaucracy can record their deaths.

The result is an almost certain discrepancy between confirmed (i.e., officially registered) deaths and actual deaths.

HJELMSLEV: THE LINGUISTIC SYSTEM – MODIFIED TO REFLECT FUZZINESS

'COVID-19'

EXPRESSION	→	content – 'Pathology' (evidence-based science, hoax/fake, big pharma scam, data-manipulation by governments and other agencies)
(sayability)	→	form/signified – 'Medicines' (several vaccines, Regeneron, steroids, experimental treatments still underway, medicines unavailable in many parts of the world), fake therapeutics, e.g., Trump's espousing of Clorox.
CONTENT	→	form/signifier – 'clinic', 'hospital' (National University Hospital Singapore/Mayo Clinic, rural hospitals lacking facilities in any part of the world, and so on)
(visibility)	→	content – Patients (but which ones? Donald Trump, Boris Johnson, or undiagnosed dead Covid patients in India whose bodies are being tossed into the river Ganges)

It is not being claimed here that all the concepts involved in discussing or understanding the Covid-19 pandemic are 'fuzzy'. Rather, it is the case that fuzzy concepts of the kind described here exist alongside concepts that are certainly not fuzzy. For example, it would be absurd to assume that the pharmacological science behind the development of the Covid-19 vaccines had fuzzy concepts at its core — the very success of the vaccines produced hinges on precision and accuracy, and any fuzziness that exists will be rare and overcome as soon as it is detected. Fuzziness is more likely to be found in the social and political dimensions underlying the pandemic, or in the scientific realm, in such fields as epidemiology, where the gathering of data involves a constantly moving target, and where political interference can occur at any number of points. Epidemiology is a key instrument in public health policy, and the 'outbreak analytics' it provides is vital for swift and effective responses to a disease.

Epidemiology (in particular, epidemic modelling and forecasting) is therefore crucial to understanding a disease's transmissibility, and governments may have a vested interest in concealing this transmissibility from their own citizens and also the rest of the world. Fuzziness, often in the service of government 'spin', has the opposite effect by blurring rates of transmissibility. A case in point here is the United Kingdom's government's approach to the Covid pandemic.

For all its talk of 'following the science', Boris Johnson's Conservative government adjusted epidemiological evidence to its policy preferences throughout the pandemic. Disclosure of reliable epidemiological data was delayed from the British public before being purveyed in 'massaged', and therefore often in a fuzzy or distorted, form. *The Guardian* newspaper suggests this strategy underpinned delays in UK health policy implementation:

> The delay ... helped to prime the space for private UK-based [testing] firms to enter the market. In January 2020, the UK passed on the early chance to use a viral sequence developed by a German lab and made freely available by the WHO to make a Covid test. It did, however, award last-minute public contracts for testing, tracing, and the production of PPE and ventilators to companies with little or no prior experience in similar tasks.[11]

It is clear from this and numerous other instances that governments and official agencies both lie outright about fairly conclusive epidemiological findings (no fuzziness required here!) or 'fuzzify' (pardon the neologism) the data that is available.

Evidence for the latter practice is readily available in several regions of the world. Hence, in order not to impose a general lockdown or close down schools and so forth ('we need to return to business as usual'), governments just fudge the data to declare that a 'crisis' does not yet exist.

Politically, 'crisis' must of course be one of the fuzziest concepts in existence. There were several times when the UK's Covid pandemic was at an obvious crisis point (according to distinguished epidemiologists and medical specialists), but the Tory government blithely overlooked this. By contrast, a 'crisis' is declared by the UK government (and its supporters in the right-wing tabloid media) every time a couple of dozen asylum seekers venture across the Channel from Calais in rickety dinghies and head for the English coast.

According to the BBC, as of December 2022, there were 210,000 Covid deaths in the UK. As far as we know, there have been no UK deaths caused by an asylum seeker crossing the Channel (though sinking boats have caused dozens of asylum seekers to drown).[12]

In the beginning was the political, and the political was bound to discourse.

Notes

1 Assemblages of this hybrid nature are said to embody features of the Algocene, a digitally unified world (in which there are more sensors and scanners than people!), with ever-present computerized technologies producing myriad datascapes; 'smart' products (e.g., watches which can monitor the wearer's cardiac functions, computer-based language learning); automated trading on stock

markets; regulating without human intervention supplies of electricity, water, and natural gas; surgery and bomb-disposal undertaken by robots; and so on.

2 Parts of the following section have been adapted from my work 'On Producing the Concept of the Concept-Image' (Surin 2011: 171–180).

3 The quotation from Nietzsche is in his (1968: 409). Emphases as in original.

4 In virology, the medical discourses are exemplified by putative treatments and prophylactics such as vaccines – e.g., Regeneron (at $96,000 per course of treatment, used to treat Donald Trump when he contracted Covid), and steroids such as dexamethasone (also used to treat Trump). It should be noted that there is an irreducible narrative component to concepts, so much so that it might be more accurate to use the hyphenated *narrative-concept* in place of *concept*. However, for ease of use I will continue with the latter. This narrative component can be seen when reference is made to, for example, Covid vaccines such as Pfizer, AstraZeneca, Johnson & Johnson. The concept 'Pfizer vaccine' signifies not only a small amount of liquid in a vial, but also has inserted into its signification notions of side-effects, availability, effectiveness, durability, and so forth.

5 I mention Foucault as the exemplary figure in the development of this new 'theoretics' of knowledges, but Pierre Bourdieu also did significant work in this area. The most important figure for my account, however, has been Gilles Deleuze (1986). For a more detailed treatment of the notions of concept, function, and field, see Deleuze and Guattari (1994). Deleuze has analyzed cinema as a 'crystalline regime' in his two-volume work on cinema; see also his (1966). I am deeply indebted to Deleuze's texts for my account of conceptual practice.

6 An excellent account of this distinction between the 'rational concept' and 'sensible intuition' is to be found in Levi R. Bryant (2008: 5ff). Bryant argues that Deleuze's major philosophical achievement resides in the overcoming of this age-old distinction. It is impossible to do justice to Bryant's fine book in a note, but I believe it is possible to account for the essential features of Deleuze's transcendental empiricism to be retained without taking his thought in the direction of a 'hyper-rationalism' of the kind proposed by Bryant. But there are many 'Deleuzes', and Bryant's 'Deleuze' is certainly among the more noteworthy of them – I am much indebted to his rigorous and thought-provoking book.

7 According to Deleuze, positioning something as a pure exteriority necessarily grants that pure exteriority an a priori ontological superiority over particulars since that exteriority then becomes the ground for any reflection on the character and function of the empirical particular. The function of such concepts as Being, Unity, Matter, and so forth is thus to order and group phenomena that would be disparate and unconnected if not placed 'under' these regulative concepts. 'Brute' phenomena need these regulative concepts in order to make any sense to the subject of consciousness.

8 Deleuze derives the notion that 'concepts are centers of vibrations' from Gilbert Simondon. On Simondon, see Deleuze (2005a, 2005b).

9 My understanding of fuzzy logic and fuzzy semiotics is indebted to Sangalli (1998).

10 Ian Sample, 'Covid research: Variant found in India may spread faster than type detected in Kent', *The Guardian*, May 13, 2021, https://www.theguardian.com/world/2021/may/13/uk-covid-scientists-variant-found-in-india-variant-may-be-spreading-faster-than-kent-strain.

11 Jana Bacevic and Linsey McGoey, 'The British government's Covid strategy was never designed to manage the virus' *The Guardian* (July 27, 2021), https://www.theguardian.com/commentisfree/2021/jul/27/british-government-covid-strategy-virus-incompetence-ignorance-pandemic. Accessed on February 21, 2023.

12 'Covid 19 in the UK', BBC, December 23, 2022, at https://www.bbc.com/news/uk-51768274. Accessed on February 21, 2023.

References

Bryant, Levi R. 2008. *Difference and Givenness: Deleuze's Transcendental Empiricism and the Ontology of Immanence*. Evanston: Northwestern University Press.

Deleuze, Gilles. 1966. 'Sur la régime crystallin', *Hors cadre* 4, 9–45.

Deleuze, Gilles. 1986. *Foucault*. Translated by Seán Hand. Minneapolis: University of Minnesota Press.

Deleuze, Gilles. 2005a. 'Gilbert Simondon' in David Lapoujade (ed.), *Desert Islands and Other Texts 1953–1974*, Translated by Michael Taormina, 86–89. New York: Semiotext(e).

Deleuze, Gilles. 2005b. 'The Method of Dramatization' in David Lapoujade (ed.), *Desert Islands and Other Texts 1953 1974*. Translated by Michael Taormina, 94–116. New York: Semiotext(e).

Deleuze, Gilles and Félix Guattari. 1994. *What Is Philosophy?* Translated by Hugh Tomlinson and Graham Burchell. New York: Columbia University Press.

Nietzsche, Friedrich. 1968. *The Will to Power*. Translated by Walter Kaufman and R. J. Hollingdale. New York: Vintage.

Sangalli, Arturo. 1998. *The Importance of Being Fuzzy: And Other Insights from the Border between Math and Computers*. Princeton: Princeton University Press.

Surin, Kenneth. 2011. 'On Producing the Concept of the Concept-Image' in Robert Michell and Jacques Khalip (eds.), *Releasing the Image: From Literature to New Media*, 171–180, 266–67. Palo Alto: Stanford University Press.

5

THE TIME OF UNCANNY, THE TIME OF EVENT

Daniela Angelucci

The extraordinary and difficult situation we are experiencing, due to the global spread of the coronavirus, seems to preclude the possibility of an accurate philosophical work. Until now, most intellectuals, intervening on the pandemic, have in fact given into the temptation to apply ready-made theories, or even to offer predictions about the future, sometimes tragic ones (for example, the unquestionable expansion of the "state of exception" according to Agamben (2020)), others claiming there is a change underway we should be excited about (the clear emergence of new forms of solidarity, according to Žižek (2020)). In the awareness that we are faced with a collective trauma, which like any trauma needs a long elaboration, we can try to write about it in a different way, avoiding for example any kind of prophecy. Starting from an aesthetic perspective, to be understood in a broad sense, it is perhaps possible to provide a key for interpreting the situation we have experienced and are still experiencing – the atmosphere, the images and emotions – that remains open to the traits of exceptionality and to the unexpected elements that arrive from nature and the world around us. I reiterate, however, that our present needs thought and philosophy, not a ready-made philosophy, but a thought that lets itself be surprised, impressed, and transformed by what comes "from outside". To begin with, it may be useful to quote Foucault's words, referring to Blanchot but valid for every thought that identifies in the encounters and clashes between bodies the primary cause of all events: "For us he is that thought (of the outside) itself – its real, absolutely distant, shimmering, invisible presence, its inevitable law, its calm, infinite, measured strength" (Foucault 1987: 19).

DOI: 10.4324/9781003507789-6

The Return of the Repressed

A first step we can take, then, to describe what is in many ways the traumatic experience of the virus is to recover a term proper to psychoanalysis, that of uncanny. In his 1919 essay that bears the same title, Freud (1919: 219) defined uncanny, in German *Unheimlich*, as a particular kind of fright. One must ask, however, "what this common core is which allows us to distinguish as 'uncanny' certain things which lie within the field of what is frightening" (Freud 1919: 220). Freud answers this question through an etymological analysis and a collection of examples, which however already imply a hypothesis on the meaning of the term, proposed at the beginning of the essay as a hypothesis to be verified: "I will say at once that both courses lead to the same result: the uncanny is that class of the frightening which leads back to what is known of old and long familiar" (Freud 1919: 220). Freud states that he arrived at this definition through a collection of individual cases, experiences, or impressions that evoked this particular type of fright, which were then confirmed by a linguistic study. Before moving on to the examples, he offers his reading of the etymology of the term, constructed as a negation of the adjective *heimlich*, whose first meaning is "domestic", "familiar". The root of *heimlich* is in fact the same as *Heimat*, a German noun that indicates "homeland" understood as a territory defined not by its belonging to a political system but by the bond one has with it. The first meaning of *unheimlich* is therefore "not domestic, not familiar", that is, uncanny in the sense of foreign or strange, and this is its current use. However, in his etymological research, Freud cites the German language dictionary by Daniel Sanders and notes that strangely among the various meanings of *heimlich* there is also its opposite, that which is "hidden": from the first meaning of "domestic" the meaning of the word shifts towards something intimate and therefore hidden, concealed.

To recapitulate: if *heimlich* has two meanings that are almost the opposite of each other, so will its opposite *unheimlich* have two meanings, which convey at the same time the sense of something unfamiliar but also not hidden. In short, the term *Unheimlich*, "perturbing", is constitutively twofold, and under the most obvious meaning of "foreign" hides that of "familiar". Hence the definition of Schelling, reported by Freud, who qualifies uncanny as something that should remain hidden and that instead has surfaced. The uncanny is then the return, uncontrollable and unexpected, of the repressed, according to Schelling's definition: "everything that is *unheimlich* that ought to have remained secret and hidden but has come to light" (Freud 1919: 225). Proceeding in this direction, Freud can associate the uncanny to the unconscious; he can associate the familiar strangeness of what perturbs us to the ego, defined as being no longer "master in its own house", dominated by a force that is foreign but at the same time familiar, as present and operating in our psyche.

It is no coincidence that during a radio interview given to Radio Tre's program *Uomini e profeti* (Men and Prophets) during the days of the first Italian lockdown, precisely on March 21, 2020, the psychoanalyst Manuela Fraire described the experience of the virus and the lockdown as a moment of collective psychoanalysis, a moment in which one of the great repressed elements of our society, incurable disease, the possibility of death, appeared daily before our eyes in all its evidence. The trust in science, typical of the Western mentality, evidently strong until this day even among the personalities most critical of scientism, was deeply shaken by the arrival and the consequences of the virus – it is indeed the same situation that we find ourselves in now while writing. Which is similar, and perhaps not coincidentally, to the historical moment in which Freud wrote about the uncanny, that is the terrible years of the First World War to which the author alludes *en passant*, almost shyly, apologizing for not having been able to investigate the secondary literature on the subject – in fact the reasons of this "as may easily be guessed, lie in the times in which we live" (Freud 1919: 220).

If what holds together the familiar and the foreign, the strange within the familiar is disturbing, some traits of this concept, of this atmosphere, accompany our experience of the virus, underlining its disturbing nature also because it is invisible. On the other hand, even in the course of Freudian thought itself, the hypothesis of an event that really happened, particularly in childhood, is replaced by a phantasmatic conception of trauma (Laplanche and Pontalis 2006). The threat of contagion we are learning to live with is invisible, but it exists; moreover it comes from outside, though it could also be inside me. If we are in general much more frightened by the idea of being infected by others than of being the cause of the contagion ourselves, it is more difficult to remember and accept the circumstance that we ourselves may be carrying the virus. Moving from individual denial to collective denial, we can point out how often the government authorities of many countries have emphasized the foreignness of the virus: Donald Trump has spoken insistently of a Chinese virus. It is a strategic, political, but also psychological need to place the danger outside of us, in the other. This strategy fully captures the most subtle and disturbing fear, namely that we can be carriers and not just receivers of the contagion.

The virus is both familiar and unfamiliar, the danger is us and it is others at the same time, which is the first aspect that connects our emotions and our imagination these days to the uncanny in its classic Freudian treatment. Moreover, we may be completely asymptomatic carriers of contagion, we can be unaware, guilty and innocent at the same time. Roberto De Gaetano has compared this situation to that of Sophocles' *Oedipus Rex*, who is an unconscious carrier of the plague in Thebes.

> It is a literally tragic condition that lies at the heart of the epidemic we are experiencing. It is the threatening nature of the human being that disregards all awareness and responsibility. So much so that the conductor of the contagion may be a 'healthy carrier', and therefore unaware and innocent. The potential culpability of man lies in his nature, in his very corporeity, which becomes a vehicle, a transmission, a medium of the virus.
>
> *(De Gaetano 2020)*

The epidemic forces us to come into contact with the body we inhabit, it prevents us from forgetting it even when it is separated from the bodies of others, in quarantine, in isolation, or when it is hidden by masks. The "guilt" of the virus ignores social positions and hierarchies, it concerns the very life that passes through us and that we are. This is precisely – literally – uncanny.

Automata and Wild Animals

But let us continue to follow Freud's text. After the etymological analysis, which emphasizes the duplicity of the uncanny, something domestic and foreign, familiar and unfamiliar, Freud's text offers a series of examples. Many of these are drawn from Hoffman's novella *The Sand-Man*, which presents a series of doubles, which can be easily connected to the experience of a foreign familiarity. Among these examples, the first – though not the most important according to Freud, who focuses on the theme of the eyes and the fear of being blinded – is that of the doll Olimpia, a creature of Dr. Spallanzani endowed with apparent life and mistaken by the protagonist of the story for the doctor's daughter, with also slightly satirical consequences. Freud cites the text of E. Jentsch, *Zur Psychologie des Unheimlichen* (1906), who reads the uncertainty about the nature of the automaton – it is not clear whether it is animate or inanimate – as a typical example of the uncanny (furthermore, the doll that comes alive is one of the topoi of horror literature and cinema).

> Jentsch has taken as a very good instance 'doubts whether an apparently animate being is really alive; or conversely, whether a lifeless object might not be in fact animate'; and he refers in this connection to the impression made by waxwork figures, ingeniously constructed dolls and automata.
>
> *(Freud 1919: 226)*

We also find this aspect in the uncertainty of the nature of the virus. As we have learned in this last year, the characteristics that distinguish a living being are not all present in the organization of viruses, which, although they are biological entities, do not have their own metabolism and cannot grow and multiply independently. Not being able to define them as "living organisms", we adopt the expression "parasites". The virus is made of life, of DNA, but it does not live on its own, it needs to be "carried" by others. In short, it has an uncertain nature; it is alive and not alive at the same time. This aspect is echoed in the words of Žižek (2020):

> What we should accept and reconcile ourselves to, is that there is a sub-layer of life, the undead, stupidly repetitive, pre-sexual life of viruses, which has always been there and which will always be with us as a dark shadow, posing a threat to our very survival, exploding when we least expect it.

If the virus is life and it is "always with us", if it is part of human nature in its corporeity, guilty and innocent at the same time, it is possible that in this uncanny experience, as in all human experiences, there is the possibility of a recognition, an elaboration, and perhaps even an opportunity.

The duplicity of the uncanny, its characteristic of being both familiar and unfamiliar, fits not only with the invisible presence of the virus in our lives but also with the transformation that places have undergone as a result of this presence. This element of disorientation also appears in the Freudian writing as an example of the uncanny. Freud recounts his personal experience of loss of orientation, precisely in an Italian town: the unintentional return to the same places and the consequent dual sensation of recognition and estrangement produce in him a feeling of perturbing powerlessness. Such disruption may perhaps also qualify how we have experienced the emptied and transformed cities during the lockdown. Many articles in newspapers and magazines have highlighted the return to cities of some species of birds, of wild animals no longer disturbed by traffic and noise, therefore present at unusual times and places (Singh 2020). This new presence is enough to change our gaze on the places we inhabit, to relocate the category of urban and to understand it no longer as separate from nature, but also to change the way we look at ourselves, if it is true that our fate appears so intertwined with that of non-human living beings (the virus itself should have been enough to teach us this). Our cities have emptied and filled with different presences; they have become quieter, less inhabited, darker. The photos of Rome, the city where I live, in the days of the March 2020 lockdown, but also the emptied historic center of the city in the following months, show very beautiful and also disturbing views: the deserted city, the same but different, familiar but foreign, seems to hide an invisible danger and at the same time appears poignantly beautiful.

The Perturbing on the Surface

Starting from the uncertain nature of the virus, from its being therefore literally perturbing – that is, inside and outside at the same time, familiar and unknown at the same time, alive and not alive at the same time – it is then possible to link it to the Deleuzian theme of the event, as elaborated in various texts, but especially in *Logic of Sense* (Deleuze 1990). As is well known, in the texts written together with Guattari, Deleuze carried out a fierce critique of psychoanalysis, especially of its function of normalization and control. But we also know that his work is imbued with psychoanalytic elements, and that he himself would criticize his book *Logic of Sense* because it was still too benevolent towards psychoanalysis (Abou-Rihan 2008). However, I do not want to deal with the proximities and differences between Deleuze and psychoanalysis, but rather to reason on the fact that the uncanny nature of the virus – its being double, inside and outside – and above all the experience that we have had and have of it allows us to speak of it as an event in the Deleuzian sense.

We can define *Logic of Sense* as the text in which Deleuze proposes a thought of surfaces, rejecting dualism in an ontological sense (against transcendence), in a logical sense (against representation), and in an ethical sense (against the transcendent norm). In his effort to overthrow Platonism, in addition to using the work of Lewis Carroll and many other authors, Deleuze (1990: 4) calls into question the Stoics, who oppose a worldview in which everything is a mixture of bodies to the Platonic theory of the relationship between ideas and the sensory world. "First, there are bodies with their tensions, physical qualities, actions and passions, and the corresponding 'states of affairs'. These states of affairs, actions and passions, are determined by the mixtures of bodies". Deleuze takes up Stoic materialism in order to overthrow Platonism, since this view displaces any principle of organization: the clash and encounter between bodies in fact provides an unorganized mixture, not reducible to rules or to unity.

How then does the concept of event emerge from this materialism? The event serves to preserve the need for meaning, for something that goes beyond raw materialism: the event is the attempt to place the idea not in the hyperuranion but on the surface, on the plane of immanence. There are bodies which are causes, and then there are the effects of these causes, which are events, which are incorporeal but caused by bodies and inseparable from them.

> Second, all bodies are causes in relation to each other, and causes for each other – but causes of what? They are causes of certain things of entirely different nature. These effects are not bodies, but properly speaking incorporeal entities. [...] They are not things or facts, but events.
>
> *(Ibid.: 4–5)*

In this perspective the first causes are not ideas, but bodies, of which incorporeal events are surface effects, different in nature from bodies, but inseparable from them as the fog rising from a prairie is inseparable. Between bodies and incorporeal events there is no separation, although the event is not confused with the body as its effect is.

In other words, we must therefore distinguish between event and happening, although the two are not concretely separable. Happening is the encounter between bodies, that is, the spatio-temporal realization, the state of affairs, while event is its incorporeal double, the effect and sense of happening. What is the relationship between bodies and event? The event is like a vapor that surrounds bodies, different in nature from corporeality but inseparable from it. The platonic idea stands out on a supersensible plane, separated from the sensible world, while the event is an effect of bodily states that is not corporeal but inseparable from the body itself, and that has a different temporality from the linear, chronological time of facts. It is an absolute becoming that acquires a strange temporality. Sense, different from the material encounters between bodies, is therefore produced by matter in the randomness of encounters. "What was eluding the Idea climbed up to the surface, that is the incorporeal limit, and represents now all possible *ideality*, the latter being stripped of its causal and spiritual efficacy. The Stoics discovered surface effects" (Deleuze 1990: 7). With a historical-philosophical operation typical of his way of thinking, by recovering and manipulating Stoic philosophy with a strange kind of faithful infidelity, Deleuze preserves the need for a sense that goes beyond matter without denying matter itself, without reintroducing transcendence. The event is what allows us to maintain the materialist line from which I started, which does not renounce the "passion for the outside", for the events that affect us coming from outside, from the natural world, from non-human living beings, without, however, denying the need to make these events – already uncanny in themselves – an experience of meaning.

James Williams (2005: 154), in his book commentary on *Difference and Repetition*, states that "for Deleuze, an event is more of the order of the uncanny connection than the essential internal truth." In fact, it is about changing intensities like "the bubbling up of animal passions in a riot". It is

> also of the order of the anomaly associated with a scientific paradigm shift or an unexpected turn in evolution. ... Instead, events, as anomalies or mutations, are distant and hard to digest occurrences requiring shifts in our established forms of knowledge or ways of thinking.

Williams continues:

> But it is important to view paradigm shifts in science or evolutionary jumps as cases that reveal something about Deleuze's events rather than as the sole or main type of event. The event has to be individual, in the sense where a sensation within an individual is the sign of an ideal event. So the shift from one set of scientific laws to another is not the event, neither is

> the emergence of a new species. The event is the first sign of mutation or the first sensation that something anomalous is significant (in a scientist, a spectator, an actor, animal, plant or molecule).
>
> *(Williams 2005: 154)*

The Truth of the Virus

The uncertain nature of the virus, its invisibility, its difficult location, its perturbing being, alive and dead at the same time, already leads us towards an uncertain ontology, which welcomes the outside, nature, the matter indifferent to the human, but also captures the inseparability with its expressions, with its sense. Searching for the sense of this happening that we have witnessed and are still witnessing as a product of encounters and clashes between bodies, between different species, means experiencing it, grasping it as an event from which perhaps we can learn something.

First of all, it is perhaps necessary to explicate the fact that despite the obviousness of what I am writing, nothing like the unexpected arrival of an invisible virus, which proliferates thanks to our metabolism, teaches us the power of nature and the inseparability of sense, expression, of the incorporeal, from matter. What it teaches us, in short, is a thought of immanence. Secondly – this is not a very original statement, but it is worth repeating – the current situation forces us to abandon the traditional idea of separation (and hierarchy) between species. Here it is worth quoting the words of Gilles Deleuze and Félix Guattari about viruses and the conceptual invention of the rhizome in the introduction of the book *A Thousand Plateaus*, despite the fact they are already much quoted in this period. The description of the rhizome, a botanical term that the two authors borrow to describe a model of being and thinking that is multiple and made of infinite connections, as opposed to the classical, organic model based on binary logic, is in fact very well suited to a situation in which the central position of the human being in the world is being questioned.

> We form a rhizome with our viruses, or rather our viruses cause us to form a rhizome with other animals. [...] Transversal communications between different lines scramble the genealogical trees. Always look for the molecular, or even submolecular, particle with which we are allied. We evolve and die more from our polymorphous and rhizomatic flus than from hereditary diseases, or diseases that have their own line of descent. The rhizome is an anti-genealogy.
>
> *(Deleuze and Guattari 2005: 11)*

The power of nature and the inseparability of the human being from other species are two aspects highlighted by the current situation widely emphasized by many commentators, journalists, and philosophers (Solnit 2020).[1] But what I would like to emphasize most here is that talking about the virus as an event in the Deleuzian sense, and precisely as a perturbing event, trains us to always keep in mind the disturbing aspect of a materialist thought. The thought of immanence is optimistic, although its optimism is of a desperate kind, since it is constituted in the confrontation with what resists in the face of thought. The Deleuzian idea of life as a clash of bodies and as a continuous metamorphosis – of which the virus was an obvious example for Deleuze and Guattari as early as 1980 – is at the same time liberating and aggressive, transformative and frightening.[2]

The latest book by Emanuele Coccia (2021), entitled *Métamorphosis*, by describing every birth as an occupation of another body, every life as a relationship with a multiplicity of other forms, every species as a *mélange* of other species, shows – perhaps even beyond the author's intentions – how life itself is disturbing and ambiguous. All living forms are capable of imposing a new order, a new perspective, a new way of existing, but in every opening to the unprecedented there is a disturbing, obscure and destructive part, which must be thought, put into play and questioned, even when taken as a possibility for change. This is the meaning of *Amor fati*, also at the center of the book *Logic of Sense* in its undeniable Nietzschean inspiration: often the event, writes Deleuze (1990: 151) himself, is "a kind of plague, war, wound or death", but wanting the event doesn't mean resigning, as much as it does "to release its eternal truth", wanting "not exactly what occurs, but something in that which occurs" (Deleuze 1990: 149).

Notes

1 From a more theoretical perspective, for a connection between the virus and contemporary materialist thought see T. Sikka, "Feminist Materialism and Covid-19: The Agential Activation of Everyday Objects", *Nordic Journal of Feminist and Gender Research*, 2021, 21, pp. 4–16.

2 Despite all the differences between the two perspectives, it is worth remembering that in his most difficult and mysterious book, *Beyond the Pleasure Principle*, Freud also proposed the thesis of the inseparability of eros and thanatos.

Bibliography

Abou-Rihan, Fadi. 2008. *Deleuze and Guattari. A Psychoanalytic Itinerary*. London: Continuum.

Agamben, Georgio. 2020. *The Invention of an Epidemic*. https://www.quodlibet.it/giorgio-agamben-l-invenzione-di-un-epidemia), transl. in "European Journal of Psychoanalysis", https://www.journal-psychoanalysis.eu/coronavirus-and-philosophers/ (accessed on 26 February 2020).

Coccia, Emanuele. 2021. *Metamorphoses*. Cambridge: Polity Press.

De Gaetano, Roberto. 2020 *Il trauma del virus*, Fata Morgana web, https://www.fatamorganaweb.it/il-trauma-del-virus/ (accessed on 22 March 2020).

Deleuze, Gilles. 1990. *Logic of Sense*. Trans. Constantin V. Boundas. London: The Athlone Press.
Deleuze, Gilles and Felix Guattari. 2005. *A Thousand Plateaus. Capitalism and Schizophrenia*, Trans. Brian Massumi. London: Minnesota Press.
Foucault, Michel. 1987. Maurice Blanchot: The Thought from Outside, in *Foucault/Blanchot*, pp. 9–58. Transl. Brian Massumi. New York: Zone Books.
Freud, Sigmund. 1919. The "Uncanny", in J. Strachet (ed.), *The Standard Edition of the Complete Psychological Works of Sigmund Freud*, vol. XVII. London: The Hogart Press.
Laplanche, J. and J.-B. Pontalis. 2006. *The Language of Psychoanalysis*. New York: Routledge.
Sikka, Tina. 2021. Feminist Materialism and Covid-19: The Agential Activation of Everyday Objects, *Nordic Journal of Feminist and Gender Research*, 21, 4–16.
Singh, M. 2020. "Emboldened Wild Animals Venture into Locked-Down Cities Worldwide", *The Guardian*, https://www.theguardian.com/world/2020/mar/22/animals-cities-coronavirus-lockdowns-deer-raccoons/
Solnit, R. 2020. "What Coronavirus Can Teach Us About Hope", *The Guardian*, 7 April 2020, https://www.theguardian.com/world/2020/apr/07/what-coronavirus-can-teach-us-about-hope-rebecca-solnit (accessed on 7 April 2020).
Williams, James. 2005. *Gilles Deleuze's Difference and Repetition. A Critical Introduction and Guide*, Edinburgh: Edinburgh University Press.
Žižek, Slavoj. 2020. *Pan(dem)ic!: COVID-19 Shakes the World*, New York, London: OR Books.

PART II

Politics of the Pandemic

6

COVID-19 AND THE PRODUCTION OF KNOWLEDGE

Communication, Control, and the Citizenry

Saima Saeed

Introduction

The production and circulation of information on COVID-19 has no parallel in human history. Never before were 7.8 billion people on the planet subject to a simultaneous and extensive 'infodemic' (in World Health Organization's parlance) of this volume in the name of controlling the pandemic. The scientific rationale justifying global surveillance and nation-states' attempts at gaining control over individuals and their biomedical conditions create new regimes of control and power mediated through hegemonic and statist news communication networks and technologies. They exemplify expansive forms of data surveillance in the name of health securitisation, producing outcomes that are contrary to advancing democratic values, social equity, and justice among populations.

The SARS-CoV-2 virus and its disease COVID-19 that resulted in the global pandemic since March 2020 differs from other pandemics known so far, such as SARS, zika, swine flu, and ebola in two ways: First, in its news narrativisation which has been carried out through a complex matrix of algorithmic data empiricism, numbers, and computed projections and predictions about the future 'waves'. The second point of difference is how this data is used by governments, with active corroboration of the media, to justify widespread curtailment of liberties and restrictions on public life. Such a massive mathematisation of the entire world's population into COVID 'positive', 'negative', and 'recovered' categories far surpasses the earlier known panoptic mechanisms of observing, spatialising, and regulating populations, in both its scale and social and psychological impact. Such categorisation plays a key role in the cognitive bridging of the mathematical data to the level

DOI: 10.4324/9781003507789-8

of the everyday, presented by the news media in diurnal, even hourly cycles of fresh infectivity, transmission, and news about new variants. The pandemic dataset – national and global – is collated, circulated, and refreshed every day with remarkable alacrity and serialisation. Social media platforms bombard messages that advise a total withdrawal from anything social, as ill-prepared governments with poor health infrastructure and multinational organisations and corporations devise novel ways to profit from the global health crisis.

The paper is divided into two parts that address these two related aspects of the pandemic under investigation – one, the epistemological question of the nature of news and knowledge production about the pandemic. The second is locating the political, economic, and technological dynamics that have led to the first and contributed to the production of an 'infodemic' whose most telling consequences have been the disempowering of citizens and decline in trust in democratic institutions and media, thereby resulting in an overall weakening of democracies.

Part I

The Pandemic News: Epidemiological Data and Its Epistemological Considerations

The pandemic has occasioned a scrutiny of the epistemic basis of the information on which rests all labels, meaning, and language that make the COVID-19 pandemic, a pandemic. The 24/7 inundation of COVID news, especially through internet-driven social media platforms like Twitter that Hermida (2010) aptly describes as 'ambient journalism', are characterized as 'always-on communication systems', resulting in an ecosystem of multiple and asynchronous media narratives that are received, exchanged, and broadcast all at once to a global audience. This is also the reason that makes COVID-19 the first pandemic where studying the virus and its replication is as definitive to the disease as how it is understood and narrated to the world's population. Ironically, early enough in the pandemic timeline, it was the WHO itself that blew the whistle on the magnitude of the crisis that was going to befall upon a hapless world population with *warnings of not one but two pandemics simultaneously – one biological, the other informational, one a pandemic and the other an 'infodemic'*.

Anticipating this, WHO had a month prior to declaring COVID-19 a pandemic in its press briefing on March 11, 2020, warned of an 'infodemic' in its Situation Report-13 issued on the worldwide data of confirmed cases of 2019-nCoV as on February 2, 2020. The report defined what WHO meant by an infodemic and how its risk communications and social media teams were working 24/7 to bust myths and rumors that could potentially be harmful to the health of the public. In particular, it referred to how it would use social media platforms and media channels including Facebook, Instagram, Twitter, LinkedIn, and Weibo to counter the infodemic, which it defined as 'an over-abundance of information – some accurate and some not – that makes it hard for people to find trustworthy sources and reliable guidance when they need it' (WHO website 2021).[1] The WHO toolkit enlisting ways to fight the infodemic points to a more dreaded enemy – hate speech and its polarizing potential to swing the COVID public discourse that would hold dangerous consequences for human rights and the future of democracies.[2]

At the World Health Assembly in May 2020, WHO member states passed Resolution WHA73.1 on the COVID-19 response. The resolution recognizes that managing the infodemic is a critical part of controlling the COVID-19 pandemic. It calls on member states to provide reliable COVID-19 content, take measures to counter misinformation and disinformation, and leverage digital technologies across the response. WHO's website maintains a separate page on 'risk communication' that specifically addresses the issue of 'infodemic management'[3] which the multilateral agency defines as 'applying evidence-based interventions that bring understandable, localized evidence-based information to citizens and drive positive health-seeking behaviour'. (WHO Website 2021).[4]

Caught in the slippery lattices of the COVID infodemic are citizen-subjects whose cognitive and affective ability to rationalise and independently test the validity of information being circulated is systematically blunted. Even if we were to set the 'infodemic' aside, the epistemic basis of our knowledge about SARS-CoV-2 virus and its disease COVID, largely mediated through the news media, necessitates *a critical re-thinking about the nature of news itself. News reporters are not scientists, and neither is journalism science.* Given the journalistic tendency of oversimplification, subjectivation, and ideological impregnation that are inherent to the process of news production, it is surmised that media lack the language to represent science. Is a selective production of scientific knowledge as practiced by the media untrustworthy? Does such a selection influence how science is narrated, received, and understood by the ordinary public? A large volume of work disputing the objectivity claims of the Anglo-American tradition of news making, specifically those that point to the politics of sourcing of information (Gans 1979) 'social production of news' (Hall et al. 1978: 53–60), the politics of its narrative form (Schudson 1995), the agenda-setting function of mass media (McCombs and Shaw 1972), and 'framing' as inherent to the news production process (Entman 1993 Eveland 2004; Goffman 1974) point to the constructivist nature of the news text. In the case of the COVID-19 pandemic, this subjectivity of the news making process was most readily exploited by governments with ill-prepared health systems to hide their handling of the pandemic, on the one hand, and by 'organized crime elements, conspiracy theorists, anti-vaxxers, and anarchist groups that have an interest in undermining confidence in the medical and political establishment' (Schulman and Siman-Tov 2020: 2), on the other, leading to opposing ideas particularly around vaccination and its efficacy and after-effects.

In the report, Schulman and Siman-Tov recommended the urgent stipulation to 'increase public awareness of the need to reduce the contamination of the discourse about the pandemic' (2020: 4) through launch of technological tools to detect content that is manipulated, bots, and fake websites. Besides, it calls for the establishment of a designated and integrated organization that focuses on cooperation between the relevant government ministries and civil society organizations, including media outlets and research institutes (Schulman and Siman-Tov 2020: 5). Information manipulation is an aspect of the infodemic that poses serious consequences for the pandemic response, mitigation, and preparedness and the overall public health policy outcome. Much of the botched government response is attributed to information chaos due to manipulative framing of the pandemic and suppression of information.

Kovalčíková and Tabatabai (2020) argue that despite the differences in their audiences and interests, authoritarian regimes shared the following five common messaging frames that helped enhance each other's information manipulation efforts: rehabilitating China's image, questioning the origin of the virus, shifting the blame to U.S. sanctions with hash tags like #medicalterrorism, highlighting failures in democracies, and finally promotion of authoritarianism over democracies. Public trust in democratic institutions, facts, and data is undermined as authoritarian governments utilized the opportunities presented to them by this global public-health crisis that continued unabated till 2022.

Coronavirus news draws heavily from the effect that visual depictions of the virus generate, an unqualified fear from the spiked, corona crown protein cover. The viral is universal not just in the biotic fact of it being a geographically omnipotent and spreadable virus but also by the verity that the abstraction is buttressed by the concrete visual representation of it in news stories that use high-end graphics and symbolism to represent a scientific phenomenon or species which the news text is neither capable of verifying independently nor articulating fully. Yet the news narrative relies heavily on classifications and the given grids of meanings like the typology of dividing the country populations into 'positive', 'negative', and 'recovered' as received data that is faithfully reproduced in terms of screen graphics and reinforced by sound bites and live interviews of institutional and legitimized sources like those of the WHO chief, heads of states, health ministry statements of different nations, and approved 'COVID experts' on prime time television channels. Moreover, the diurnal nature of this daily count of COVID cases across nations perfectly suits the news narrative's own format that feeds on a 24/7 news cycle of production and circulation. The volume of it can be estimated by the fact that by October 15, 2020, the word 'COVID-19' yielded about 608,000,0000 results on Google while a search with the name 'coronavirus' yielded approximately 2,770,000,000 results on the same search engine giant.

The methodological imperative of COVID-19's empirico-hypothetico-deductive reordering and classification of the world's population is contingent on a news narrative format that draws from what Robert E. Park referred to as its 'transient and ephemeral quality' (1940: 676) in a critical essay on 'news as a form of knowledge'. In country after country, the citizen subject was bombarded by competing and contradictory sets of information wherein the recommendations made by the public health officials like those around wearing masks were negated by influential figures, including delayed responses by heads of states like Justin Trudeau and Donald Trump. The pandemic communication has been marked by polarized debates on the efficacy of masks to prevent the spread of the contagion or even of the vaccine to protect against contracting the disease in future. In the lack of clear scientific evidence-based data bolstered by beguiling media narratives that played a huge part in spreading disinformation in violation of journalistic principles and ethics, scholars point out how public health officials like Fauci lost public support and credibility (Smith and Wanless 2020). Referring to Trump's anti-Fauci retweet that read, 'Sorry Fake News, it's all on tape...', Smith and Wanless (2020) state that 'The United States demonstrates what can happen when there is disunity, disinformation, and inconsistency in official messaging in a crisis situation' (2020: 7). A similar polarization of opinion was seen in the Canadian media when the Canadian prime minister was attacked by the opposition for following the advice of Dr. Theresa Tam, a leading Canadian doctor, too closely. A few far-right media organizations started a petition to get Dr Tam fired and managed to collect 40,000 signatures in two weeks (Smith and Wanless 2020: 7).

Reporting Science and Medicine: The Subjectivisation of Objective Knowledge

Weber (1949) posits the issue of the application of 'general objectively valid truth' to those disciplines which are concerned with social and cultural phenomena (Weber 1949: 51). Weber therefore points to the need to (1) differentiate between 'existential knowledge', that is, knowledge of what is, from the knowledge of what ought to be, or 'normative knowledge' (Weber 1949: 51); and (2) the need to take into cognizance the means of inquiring and not just its end (Weber 1949: 52), making the question of appropriateness of means or method critical to inquiry itself. This is especially important in regard to social policy that is based on scientific knowledge. Weber regarded the particular/concrete/specific as a 'value relevant' phenomenon for which social scientists must have adequately justifiable and appropriate explanation.

A Weberian understanding of the relationship between concept and reality of the coronavirus, that is, between the idea and the 'ideal-type' (Weber 1949: 95–98), entails two different sets of methodological approaches and theoretical suppositions about the virus:

1. as a biological entity – empirical reality that lays claim to an empirical truth – and
2. as a sociological, psychological, economic, and philosophical concept – analytical aspects that are contingent on value judgments

News reporters by the virtue of their professional training and given the values in news (intrinsic, professional, and ideological) are suited to deal with the latter while the former belongs to the domain of scientists and researchers in the natural sciences. However, this neat categorisation is clearly breached when it comes to science, health, and medical reportage. The choice of 'experts' and 'doctors' to fill in for this technical (read science and medicinal) information is always a subjective one for the media organization. It is neither apolitical nor 'objective' as it does not bracket out differences that arise out of the nationality, race, affiliation, and class of the 'expert'. Such a journalistic selection of who is entitled to speak about the pandemic and the granting of legitimacy thereof to a few such actors and agencies not only fails to bridge the severe class and gender divide that the pandemic created but ends up reinforcing them, evident in the differential pandemic responses of the rich and poor, women and vulnerable populations. This also points to another methodological consideration, namely that despite the universality of the empirical biological entity and its presence, the specificity of its experience and impact on life have to be understood, investigated, and reported at the individual, group, community, and national levels. This again reiterates that neither are journalists scientists nor is news-making devoid of value judgments and ethical concerns about how empirical truths are determined and represented in news.

Badiou (2005) relates the dialectics of knowledge/truth to 'post-evental fidelity' (2005: 331) and the ontological differentiation between the true and the veridical. Knowledge for him is the capacity to discern multiples within a situation and is oriented to discernment (presentation), whereas classification concerns the connection between language and a part of the situation, the multiples of multiples, and therefore it is oriented towards representation (Badiou 2005: 328). Badiou distinguishes between fact and 'event' in terms of their origin from a local (*in-situ*) site from where the event first emerges and to which the situation can be historically related, as truth originates there. For the coronavirus pandemic it was Wuhan, China in December 2019.

The event presents a 'plenitude of multiples', and that for Badiou constitutes the truth procedure that is contained in the being in his expression, 'Being qua being is thus doubly submitted to nominations and explanations' (Badiou 2005: 316).

Between Presentation and Representation: Veracity and Sourcing in the News Text

An analysis of the COVID-19 pandemic in a Badiousian sense of all situations being structured-twice, entailing presentation and representation (Badiou 2005: 94), reveals that *the pandemic is more represented than presented by the media, both in the volume and nature of its reportage, for reasons of the State*. To recall the three possibilities in the presentation–representation spectrum, *normal* (that which is both presented and represented), *excrescence* (that which is only represented but not presented) and *singular* (when only presented but not represented) as Badiou (2005: 99) sees them, the state manifests excrescence, the proletariat is a singular, whereas the bourgeoisie is a normal term being presented economically and represented by the State (2005: 109). A COVID-19 pandemic example of the gap between presentation and representation is the huge mismatch between the reported COVID deaths and the actual deaths as it has emerged in the WHO report published in May 2022. The WHO 'excess mortality' report (WHO 2022) based on a methodology developed by their Technical Advisory Group for COVID-19 Mortality Assessment and country consultations, released on May 5, 2022, estimated that the COVID pandemic caused 14.91 million deaths, whereas it was hugely underreported to only 5.42 million. The realization that the reported figures were 2.7 times lesser than the actual shocked the world.

The report points out that 68 percent of excess deaths are concentrated in just 10 countries globally. Like with many other countries, India too underreported its data. WHO data reveals that India reported 481,000 Covid deaths between January 1, 2020 and December 31, 2021, which were alarmingly 10 times lesser than the figures that were put out by WHO, establishing that India accounted for nearly a third of Covid deaths globally.[5]

A socio-political appraisal of the policies and legislation related to the pandemic in most countries (for instance, in India various curbs were invoked under the enforcement of the Disaster Management Act) reveals the workings of '*positivist* epistemologies and *programmatic* politics' (Badiou 2005: 291, emphasis in original). Badiou's contention that 'positivism renders science a matter of the state' (2005: 292) is nowhere more vindicated than during the 2020 pandemic with its data about the contagion and vaccination being controlled through centralized laboratories and agencies of various governments at national levels and globally by the WHO. Health reporting, and more specifically, as in the instance of the WHO report discussed previously, death is not an independent event that is intrinsically newsworthy but a matter of the State. This language of narrating the pandemic in terms of epistemologies, mathematical modeling, data analytics, and predictions of 'waves' is the language of politics used within the metastructural field of the State or external agencies like the WHO speaking on a global level. And as Badiou explains further, positivism renders science a matter of the State by giving legal status to 'testimonials, experiments and statistics' (Badiou 2005: 292) such as mandatory vaccination certificates at the airports and statistics that countries use to justify sealing off of borders and airports from countries that report high corona positivity rate. Therefore, Badiou's conclusion that 'the positivist is a professional in the maintenance of the apparatuses of discernment' (Badiou 2005: 292) makes data scientists and journalists equally complicit in this fabrication, the former by a deft play of numbers and the latter by their use of language and selective reportage. Journalism systematically categorizes and compresses the multiples that an event presents to maintain the State and its control over the population. *Media's loyalty thus accrues to political and corporate power and their maintenance and not to the citizens whose world it orders through information management.*

Three significant questions that arise are–Do the news media have the epistemological 'fidelity' to deal with global events of this nature and scale? And, what is the 'truth procedure' that journalists employ when reporting on matters of health and science? Are the narrative structure and temporality of the news ill suited to establishing any long-term ethical fidelity to an event to present its reality in all its multiples? It is useful to turn to Robert Ezra Park who as early as 1940, examining the question of 'news as a form of knowledge', distinguishes it from history and other disciplines in its lack of such fidelity. Park states,

> News is not history because, for one thing among others, it deals, on the whole, with isolated events and does not seek to relate them to one another either in the form of causal or in the form of teleological sequences. History not only describes events but seeks to put them in their proper place in the historical succession. ... On the other hand, a reporter, as distinguished from a historian, seeks merely to record each single event as it occurs and is concerned with the past and future only in so far as these throw light on what is actual and present.
>
> *(Park 1940: 675)*

The essentially 'transient and ephemeral' quality of news (Park 1940: 676) disqualifies it from any philosophical, historical, and reflexive understanding of an event and from the formation of knowledge as he further explains: 'News, as a form of knowledge, is not primarily concerned either with the past or with the future but rather with the present' (*Ibid.*: 676) and therefore is a 'cold fact' (Park 1940). News, therefore, does not have the ethical fidelity and procedural truthfulness that history or philosophy demonstrate. Despite such a lack, it plays a key role in initiating and disseminating first information about an event to the public. It serves as a precursor and a catalyst and then abandons the project halfway. Moreover, its commitment lies with the capitalist system that funds its production and not the public which is the recipient of the news stories. This necessitates that the media imbue one meaning to the event that is dictated by such partisan interests. Such flattening of meaning comes in the way of multiplicity and plurality of information, which are presuppositions for a critical public sphere as Habermas enunciated in *The Structural Transformation of the Public Sphere* (1989). This then leads to part II of this paper that maps such imperatives in their structural setting of the State, market, and the media during a public health emergency.

Part II

Surveillance, Social Control, and the State's Politico-Medical Imperatives

The pandemic has reinforced the profit–loss calculus of capitalist societies where vaccine wars along with surveillance capitalism have bared the ruthless side of market economies exacerbated by ill-prepared states with poor health systems, triggering the rise of algorithm-based big data surveillance to predict outcomes like future waves and justify stringent curbs on democratic rights. However, the universalist and collectivist drive for vaccination is nonetheless administrable only on an individualised self of singular bodies. It is worth recalling the debates when the first vaccines were invented. Vaccination was understood as a private enterprise and a first step into the 'medicalisation of individuals' (Foucault 1980: 174–75) emanating from 'a family-children complex' (*Ibid.*) in which the family displayed the private ethic of good health and hygiene by getting the children vaccinated. Since the COVID pandemic, vaccination has found a more powerful actor in the State through funding, production, procurement, and management of information on various vaccines, on the one hand, and by controlling and monitoring the administration of the same, on the other.

Many states like India controlled the COVID vaccination of their population, making it mandatory for citizens to register for vaccination through a centrally managed and monitored portal that records the exact date, time, and venue of the vaccination and also issues a certificate for future use and reference. This interventionist, regulated institutionalisation of vaccination of the population accrues tremendous power and moral standing to the benevolent State over its citizens' wellbeing as it claims to know what is in their best interest with massive media campaigns to support such claims.

Most states have displayed this normative role of being the chief benefactor and patron watching over the interest of its citizens even as they create fresh marginalities with poor, vulnerable, and migrant populations left out of such drives. However, the benevolence of the State comes at a cost, the price being personal freedom with media narratives justifying and legitimising the sanctioning of such authoritarian interventions. Sociologist David Lyon (2021) draws attention to what he calls 'pandemic surveillance', a rampant phenomenon of watching populations routinely in their everyday lives through 'tech solutionism' using expansive technological infrastructure and digital platforms even as citizens are unaware of being watched. Pandemic surveillance therefore entails purposeful, systematic, and routine observation and attention to personal details using digital data such that public health surveillance, in particular, would be made available to law enforcing agencies for disease prevention and control (Lyon 2021). Zuboff's 'surveillance capitalism' (2019), which works by 'kidnapping human experience' through a maze of extraction and prediction imperatives, has since the COVID pandemic found a new avatar in biomedical and pharmaceutical corporations. Top biopharmaceutical companies and vaccine manufacturers of the world like Pfizer, Moderna, and Johnson & Johnson saw national governments queuing up for booking vaccines in advance, resulting in 'vaccine nationalism' wherein began an unstated race among nations to have larger number of vaccinated citizens with monetisation, funding, and politics of regulatory approvals hidden behind the overt and covert contest to save the world. As Zuboff (2019) sums up succinctly,

> Surveillance capitalism operates through unprecedented asymmetries in knowledge and the power that accrues to knowledge. Surveillance capitalists know everything about us, whereas their operations are designed to be unknowable to us. They accumulate vast domains of new knowledge from us, but not for us. They predict our futures for the sake of others' gain, not ours.
>
> *(2019: 17–18)*

Under the scepter of the pandemic, the rights and duties of the citizen were redefined by the administrative machinery of the State with hospitals and media playing key roles in this altered landscape (Figure 6.1). This complex interplay between the different institutions and stakeholders that shaped the pandemic is depicted in the form of a *closed polygon.*

In the figure, the following five vertices of the polygon are seen as the main drivers of our everyday experience of the COVID-19 pandemic.

1. The **State** with its regulatory mechanisms, administrative units, and legal framework institutes, authorises, legislates, and implements data surveillance

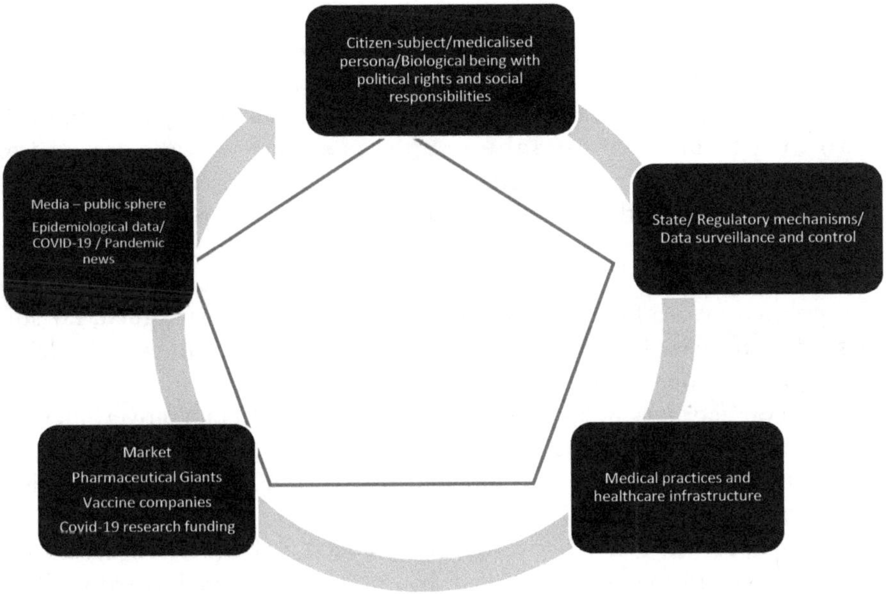

FIGURE 6.1 Revisualising the COVID-19 pandemic and its politico-medical complex.

to control the personal freedom and liberty of the citizens, through legally mandated curfews and lockdowns

2. The **healthcare infrastructure** with hospitals both public and private, prevalent medical practice, and vaccination drives shapes the disease prevention and control logic, albeit anchored under the watchful gaze of the State.
3. The **market economy** mushroomed around the healthcare sector in the wake of the pandemic with pharmaceutical giants and vaccine-related R&D laboratories funded by the State and global corporates driven by the motive to monetise and profit from the pandemic-triggered global health emergency.
4. The **media** and online platform companies not only provide legitimation for pandemic surveillance and curbing of citizens' liberties but also peddle the 'infodemic'. The political economy of such media draws from an understanding of news as a product for profit, not a service for public good. Such a paradigm does not perceive truthful information as a right that citizens are entitled to within the larger rubric of the right to information. Such loss of the ethical principle and fidelity to truth-telling due to corporatisation of the media has led to the weakening of the public sphere with telling consequences for democracies.

5. **Citizens**—the citizen with a 'medicalised persona' is the biological being who is classified as COVID positive or negative or is quarantined and on whose body the vaccine is administered. The citizen is at once the cause of the spread and also the only way to generate 'herd immunity'. The individual can't be divorced from the group even as curfews were designed to achieve such a separation. Also, policing was repurposed for surveillance that was now healthcare related and resulted in an explosion of surveillance on ordinary citizens and their biomedical parameters.

This politico-medical pentagon (a five-sided polygon), it is argued, far surpasses the concept of 'bio-politics' as enunciated by Foucault in a key delineation of relations that help locate 'governmentality', in a lecture he delivered on February 8, 1978 at College de France: 'In fact, governmentality is to the state ... what techniques of segregation [are] to psychiatry, ... techniques of discipline ... to the penal system, and biopolitics to medical institutions' (Foucault 2007: 388).

To conclude, the altered governance practiced and witnessed during the COVID-19 pandemic were marked by an unprecedented corroboration between the State, pharmaceutical giants, and technologies of surveillance refurbishing networks of control managed by an infodemic that sold the pandemic to the world's population. It breached the normative conceptualisation of information as an absolute right to becoming a partly capitalist enterprise that conceives it as a product like any other in the market. Disempowered citizens struggled to find truthful information about COVID as partisan media made no distinction between truth and misinformation.

The intent to profit from a global health crisis came to the fore during the Ebola pandemic when WHO instituted the Pandemic Emergency Financing Facility (PEF) that paved the way for the entry of private sector investment into global health. Stein and Sridhar (2017) term it as the bank's efforts to create a market for pandemic risk by marketing health as a 'global public good'. They point out that the structure of the PEF raises serious concerns as it partly works by pulling donor money away from preventing outbreaks, complicating healthcare financing and possibly overcharging donors for risk coverage operationalised by a 'two windows' structure, namely the 'insurance window' and the 'cash window' (2017: 2).

Returning to the question of knowledge production and COVID-19, the pandemic has evinced how the State's panoptic control and regulatory mechanisms including the juridical have coalesced not just with the market and AI aided data companies but with the media. Journalism, a conspicuously capitalist product since its beginnings in the nineteenth century, was zealously integrated into the network of data surveillance at a scale which is disconcerting. The questions opened up by surveillance capitalism and the use of AI for personal data aggregation for profit are no different from the warning of the refuedalisation of the media that Habermas predicted in a world before the advent of the internet. Habermas (1989: 14) locates the emergence of the 'bourgeois public sphere' to the coming of the early trade finance and trade capitalism. In this new commercial order, the '*traffic in commodities and news*' (1989: 15, emphasis in original) was an important transformation; however, it was only after the seventeenth century when news became accessible to the public that the power of the press became evident. The State soon appropriated the press as a vehicle of communicating the sovereign's ordinances and court orders to the public, using the printed word. However, the Habermasian public sphere is constituted as a push back to such a takeover by the state as a sphere that forms when 'private people come together as a public' to debate on contemporary issues that confront them. The sphere so formed is of a critical (*richtend*) public as a result of 'people's public use of their reason' (1989: 27). Ironically, it is not just that the liberty of the individual was jeopardized during the COVID-19 pandemic but that States have gotten away with severe restrictions on press freedom, controlling all news and information on the pandemic and clamping down heavily on any criticism of government health policies.

Pre-emptive of this abuse of power by nation-states, Foucault in his 1978 lectures titled '*Security, territory, population*' points to how the spatiality of the city is favorable to the spread of disease vectors, forewarning that the subject of public health will reconstitute the relations between the sovereign and the citizens in its the socio-political and juridical aspects, producing coercive forms of governmentality, an outcome that has proved prophetically true during the COVID-19 pandemic. As he explains it, 'sovereignty is exercised within the borders of a territory, discipline is exercised on the bodies of individuals, and security is exercised over a whole population' (Foucault 2007). Therefore, *surveillance, discipline*, and *control* (the three being derivative and conjugative but not interchangeable concepts in their Foucauldian usage) of the biological being is justified by modern democracies in the name of the larger interest of the health of the collectivity.

One year into the pandemic, Agamben rues that the period has generated an inordinate 'state of exception', the kind the world has not witnessed in recent history. Unprecedented as it is for the whole world to live in this state of exception at the same time, Agamben argues (2021) that such a far-reaching suspension of individual rights was not witnessed even during the two World Wars and fascism. In the February 12, 2021, entry in the *Quodlibet*, Agamben's question of 'whether governments are consciously using the pandemic to declare a "state of exception" that strengthens their powers beyond all limits or whether they have no choice but the emergency is misplaced' rings ominously pertinent. Agamben compares this 'suspension of politics' to the imposition of a framework of government that relied on 'medical terror' to consolidate its power and rule. Agamben attributes his usage of the term 'state of exception' to Carl Schmitt's *Political Theology* (1985) with its much-discussed definition of the sovereign as 'he who decides on the state of exception' (Schmitt cited in Agamben 2005). The state of exception which Agamben envisages as a 'no-man's land between public law and political fact' (Agamben 2005: 5) has a chequered history of the degree of exception, sovereign unaccountability and the nature of its imposition. It has been compared to constitutional dictatorship or a state of siege that invokes emergency measures or a suspension of law under which citizens are denied their right to resistance and basic freedoms.

Emergency provisions give extraordinary power to the State to curtail such legal provisions that make citizens sovereigns at least in matters related to their anatomical selves, that is, their own private bodies. Enforcing curfews and imposing fines for not wearing masks in public are examples of curtailment of individual freedom. However, for the first time since the Spanish flu of 1918, almost a century ago, such emergency provisions have been invoked in the domain of modern medicine and public health. As Ivan Illich (1973) had conjectured, the year 1913 was a watershed in the history of medicine not only because its effectiveness in saving lives of patients and in increasing longevity could be calibrated but also because from that point, 'new sickness was defined and institutionalized' (Illich 1973: 15), leading to the professionalisation of the 'medicine man', services, and care. Modern medicine therefore followed the trajectory of any other product of industrialisation from which the rich benefitted while the poor could not afford the costs of the 'iatrogenic diseases'. COVID-19 care and management has exhibited this symptom of what Illich called the iatrogenic or doctor-induced aberration (Illich 1973: 16), as many rich patients in the first year of the pandemic in 2020 opted to 'book' themselves a hospital bed even when they could be managed by home quarantine (convivial tool in Illich's conceptualization) and others set up oxygen cylinders at home and kept doctors as 'retainers' to meet any unforeseen emergency during the pandemic. This 'bureaucratic medicine' (Illich 1973: 17), like all other products of the post industrial society, soon spread all over the world. The pandemic proved that it was more social and behavioral aspects of the population that were instrumental in checking the spread of the contagion than medicinal intervention.

One lesson learnt from the pandemic is the ubiquitous crisis that is ensnared when unaccountable media and aberrantly institutionalised healthcare systems corroborate to produce data that drive populations into a state of fear and panic. What role should the media play during a pandemic if we are to achieve the re-tooling of society that Illich envisaged? Can we approach a reading of the news that does not dilute the epistemological question of informatisation of the citizenry under the antithetical spell of its financialisation? The question acquires greater urgency during a global health emergency like the COVID-19 pandemic which raged for over three years in varying degrees of severity. Again, we turn to Illich's call for 'demythologization of Science' (Illich 1973: 100) to stem the damage caused by it, not just for our understanding of health and education but to unpack the very nature of knowledge itself. Science for Illich was a label for a 'spectral production agency' (Illich 1973: 100) that thrives by creating a false notion of better health by its identification with institutions. Such 'institutionalization of knowledge' is delusionary as it leads to a 'paralysis of moral and political imagination' (Illich 1973: 100) since people get accustomed to having their knowledge produced for them in the form of packaged programmes and information. This in effect results in cognitive dissonance where people lose their ability to take decisions for themselves and rely on 'better knowledge' coming from elsewhere. The dependence on WhatsApp and other social media circulated fake news also stems from such a notion. The State, on its part, uses the infodemic to justify digital epidemiological tracking methods under the larger argument that technology and big data are as important in the fight against the virus as vaccines. All of these together legitimise biopolitical surveillance systems with a global footprint to which entire populations have become victims.

Conclusion

To conclude, I would like to recall a short essay by Deleuze published in 1992, where he succinctly sums up the shift from Foucault's 'disciplinary societies' to 'societies of control' (1992: 4) as a movement from a generalized crisis that environments of enclosures (analogical spaces) that prisons and hospitals invoke to the perpetual and abstract entrapments of 'control' which are 'numerical' that are 'equal to harshest of confinements' (Deleuze 1992: 4). In his oft quoted words, 'Enclosures are *molds*, distinct castings, but controls are *modulations*, like a self-deforming cast that continuously change from one moment to the other, or like a sieve whose mesh will transmute from point to point' (Deleuze 1992: 4, italics in original).

In heralding a world of corporatised healthcare systems, Deleuze warns of another more dangerous shift that is concomitant with societies of control, namely, that signatures or numbers will be replaced by 'codes', which he defines as 'the numerical language of control' that mark access to information. In the new arrangement, the individual/mass pair gives way to 'dividuals, and masses, samples, data, markets' (1992: 5). Deleuze portends that man in his new avatar of 'coded figures – deformable and transformable' (1992: 6) will bring about the most telling consequences for the Third World in a crushing form of capitalism that produces extreme poverty for three quarters of humanity (Deleuze 1992: 6). This proved to be prophetically true for the global South. The COVID-19 induced lockdown since the last week of March 2020 and intermittent lockdowns thereafter orchestrated a grave crisis for migrant workers that resulted in their mass exodus from cities and metros to their villages. Statistics revealed that during the 'second wave' of the pandemic in April–May 2021, more than 807,032 migrant workers left the capital city of Delhi for their home states in buses (*Mint* 2021). At the very least, disquieting pictures and news reports of this mass exodus laid bare the extent of the economic crisis that has gripped poor and developing nations since 2020 where the choice before the very poor has been between getting infected and food security, knowing that if coronavirus would not kill them, starvation would. Therefore, fighting COVID-19 became a relentless class question with the poor, the marginalised, and the minorities being worst affected. Yet, the corporatised media treated it as a mere human-interest story from poor nations that makes good pandemic news and refused to engage with the context in which these differences arise.

The pandemic in a cruel sense exposed the complete depoliticisation of the public sphere as a consequence of the epistemological exhaustion of news, allowing governments to become more autocratic as citizens across nations found themselves caught between a rock and a hard place in a virologically triggered global 'odyssey'.

Notes

1 https://www.who.int/teams/risk-communication/infodemic-management.
2 See WHO advisory on hate speech and COVID infodemic at https://www.who.int/news/item/23-09-2020-managing-the-covid-19-infodemic-promoting-healthy-behaviours-and-mitigating-the-harm-from-misinformation-and-disinformation Accessed on February 13, 2021.
3 See WHO's page https://www.who.int/teams/risk-communication Accessed on August 22, 2021.
4 https://www.who.int/teams/risk-communication/infodemic-management.
5 https://www.bbc.com/news/world-asia-india-60981318 Accessed May 6, 2022.

Bibliography

Agamben, Giorgio. 2005. *State of Exception.* Translated by Kevin Attell. Chicago and London: University of Chicago Press.

Agamben, Giorgio. 2021. 'The will and the necessity', *Quodlibet*, February 12, 2021.

Badiou, Alain. 2001. *Ethics: An Essay on the Understanding of Evil.* Translated by Peter Hallward. London: Verso.

Badiou, Alain. 2005. *Being and Event.* Translated by Oliver Feltham. New York: Continuum.

Deleuze, Gilles. 1992. 'Postscript on the Societies of Control', *October*, Vol. 59, 3–7.

Eveland, WP. 2004. 'The effects of political discussion in producing informed citizens: The roles of information, motivation, and elaboration'. *Political Communication*, *21*(2), 177–193.

Entman, RM. 1993. 'Framing: Towards clarification of a fractured paradigm'. *Journal of Communication*, *43*(4), 51–58.

Foucault, Michel. 1980. *Power/Knowledge: Selected Interviews and Other Writings, 1972–1977*, Colin Gordon (ed.). New York: Pantheon.

Foucault, Michel. 2007. *Security, Territory, Population: Lectures at the Collège de France, 1977-78*. Edited by Michel Senellart. Translated by Graham Burchell. New York: Palgrave Macmillan.

Gans, Herbert J. 1979. *Deciding What's News: A Study of CBS Evening News, NBC Nightly News, Newsweek, and Time*, Illinois: Northwestern University Press.

Goffman, E. 1974. *Frame Analysis: An Essay on the Organization of Experience*. New York: Harper & Row.

Habermas, Jurgen. 1989. *The Structural Transformation of the Public Sphere: An Inquiry into a Category of Bourgeois Society*. Translated by Thomas Burger, Cambridge and Massachusetts: The MIT Press.

Hermida, Alfred 2010. 'Twittering the news', *Journalism Practice*, *4*(3), 297–308.

Hall, Stuart, Chas Critcher, Tony Jefferson, John Clarke, and Brian Roberts. 1978. *Policing the Crisis: Mugging, the State and Law and Order*, London and Basingstoke: Macmillan Press Ltd.

Illich, Ivan. 1973. *Tools for Conviviality*, Glasgow: Fontana/Collins.

Lyon, David. 2021. *Pandemic Surveillance*, New Jersey: Wiley.

Kovalčíková, Nad'a and Ariane Tabatabai. 2020. 'Five Authoritarian Pandemic Messaging Frames and How to Respond', German Marshall Fund of the United States, No. 4.

Mint 2021. 'Delhi: Over 8 Lakh Migrant Workers Leave Delhi in Four Weeks of Lockdown', *The Mint*, published May 22, 2021. https://www.livemint.com/news/india/delhi-over-8-lakh-migrant-workers-leave-delhi-in-four-weeks-of-lockdown-11621676053104.html Accessed on July 5, 2021.

McCombs, Maxwell E. and Donald L. Shaw. 1972. 'The Agenda-Setting Function of Mass Media', *The Public Opinion Quarterly*, *36*(2), 176–187.

Park, Robert E. 1940. 'News as a Form of Knowledge: A Chapter in the Sociology of Knowledge', *American Journal of Sociology*, *45*(5), 669–686.

Schmitt, Carl. 1985. *Political Theology: Four Chapters on the Concept of Sovereignty*. Translated by George Schwab. Cambridge, MA: MIT Press.

Schudson, Michael. 1995. *The Power of News*, Massachusetts and London: Harvard University Press.

Schulman, R., & Siman-Tov, D. 2020. *From Biological Weapons to Miracle Drugs: Fake News about the Coronavirus Pandemic*. Institute for National Security Studies. *INSS Insights* No. 1275: 1–5.

Stein, Felix and Devi Sridhar. 2017. 'Health as a "Global Public Good": Creating a Market for Pandemic Risk', *British Medical Journal (BMJ), 358, Article j3397*, 1–4.

Smith, Victoria and Alicia Wanless. 2020. 'Public Health Experts, the Corona Virus, and the Raucous Marketplace of Ideas', Carnegie Endowment for International Peace https://www.jstor.org/stable/resrep25782.4

Weber, Max. 1949. *The Methodology of the Social Sciences*. Glencoe, IL: The Free Press.

WHO. 2022, May 5. 'Global Excess Mortality Associated with COVID-19 (Modeled Estimates)'. https://www.who.int/data/stories/global-excess-deaths-associated-with-covid-19-january-2020-december-2021 Accessed on May 6, 2022.

Zuboff, Shoshana. 2019. *The Age of Surveillance Capitalism: The Fight for a Human Future at the New Frontier of Power*. New York: Hachette Book Group.

7

PHILOSOPHY AND PANDEMICS

Agamben, Deleuze, and Zoepolitics in an Age of Covid-19

Tony See Sin Heng

Introduction

The coronavirus seems to have brought capitalism to its knees. Although the coronavirus has supposedly killed millions and disrupted various economies, it also appeared to be a global reset for a sustainable future. For once, world leaders have a rare opportunity to admit their mistakes and rethink capitalist modes of production so as to bring about a more fair, equal, and sustainable future. These initial responses were quickly dampened by the slow and sometimes dramatic realization that coronavirus might not be leaving so soon. As waves after waves of infection hit various countries at different periods with repeated mutations appearing, we slowly realized that it may not be a reset after all because there is no going back to pre-coronavirus times. Although there is much uncertainty in the midst of the coronavirus attacks, the one thing that is certain is the rise of state power. If some previously saw the rise of transnational corporations as heralding the end of the state in the 1990s, they would be greatly disappointed to say the least. For the widespread insecurity and dislocation brought about by the coronavirus infections have made the public increasingly insecure and helplessly reliant on state power. Approaching the Covid-19 crisis as an occasion for reflection on political theory, we begin with a reading of the Italian philosopher Giorgio Agamben's concept of biopolitics followed by a consideration of Deleuze and Guattari's reflection in a series of interviews about biopolitics.

Agamben and Covid-19

In a commentary on the global pandemic, Agamben (2021) reminded us that it merely accelerated the rise of biopolitics. In an interview, he states that the

DOI: 10.4324/9781003507789-9

state of exception has been used as new mode of governance, a way of militarizing public hygiene to secure control. 'Such a vague and undetermined definition will make it possible to rapidly extend the state of exception to all regions, as it's almost impossible that other such cases will not appear elsewhere' (Agamben 2020: 1). In other words, while we should be worried about being infected by the virus and its damage, we should also be worried about the quiet rise of the state form through the introduction of what he calls the 'state of exception' as the new norm in politics (Agamben 2020: 1). This is the reason why at this juncture, states would intensify the fear and insecurity associated with the virus, while leaving the populace with little hope of security except by becoming more reliant on the state. Agamben asks 'why do the media and the authorities do their utmost to spread a state of panic, thus provoking in the authentic state of exception with serious limitations on movement and a suspension of daily life in entire regions?' (Agamben 2020: 1). Furthermore, Agamben also noted that mainstream media focused on the infection rate instead of the fatality rate of the coronavirus. The fact remains that while the infection rates are high, the actual death rate is curiously small when compared to the other conventional communicable diseases. In fact, it is less than children's death rate from annual influenza. The fact is that children die more easily from their annual influenza than from the coronavirus. Agamben states that 'In 10–15% of cases a pneumonia may develop, but one with a benign outcome in the large majority of cases. It has been estimated that only 4% of patients require intensive therapy'. When we begin to look at the scientific evidence, we see that while the virus spreads rapidly and widely, its fatality rate is much lesser than it seems. Most of those who died as a result of the virus in fact did so from some prior medical conditions. If this is so, why are governments interested in producing a general state of insecurity rather than security, sometimes incurring huge costs in economic and financial terms? Agamben believes that this is simply because the legislative decree approved by the government is nothing more than a means of exerting social control, in other words, power, over the populace (Agamben 2021). Such a vague and undetermined determination of where and when the virus would 'strike' will make it impossible to stop the state apparatus from rapidly extending its police power to all regions in the country. In short, the coronavirus opens us an opportunity for the state to extend its police power. It is one which involves the extension of the biopolitical program, making the 'state of exception' the new norm in politics.

Agamben pointed out that the biopolitical paradigm is the reason why governments the world over seem to be more interested in extending their powers of surveillance rather than adopting sensible measures to counter the rise of the pandemic. This can be seen in the excessive preoccupation with surveillance technologies, movement control, and electronic tracking devices by governments to control the spread of the disease. In fact, what we are witnessing is nothing short of increased state power into almost every area of our lives during this pandemic, through increased surveillance, drone technologies, and movement controls on the population without any sign that the disease is under control. Agamben argues that we are already living in a condition in which health has become a matter of security.

Agamben and Biopolitics

The concept of biopolitics forms the overarching theme of Agamben's oeuvre. In *Homo Sacer: Sovereign Power and Bare Life* (1998), Agamben argued that juridico-political thought in the West is inaugurated by a moment when the state removed the people from their 'political life' (*bios*), reducing them from being citizens with certain rights into 'bare life' (*zoe*). This moment created a zone of radical indistinction in which neither human nor divine laws apply to these human beings, allowing the state to exclude this group of people from any claim to political life and yet simultaneously including them within a space of political imaginary – a state of exception. The significance of this legal move is that those who were located within this space can now be killed by the state without violating any laws human or divine (Agamben 1998: 81). If this is the foundation of Western political philosophy, as Agamben argues, it also meant that Western political thought was inaugurated by a 'logic of exclusion' which operates by way of simultaneously including and excluding people from political space. This idea of biopolitics can be seen as a continuation and expansion of Foucault's 'biopolitics' in his lectures at the College de France from 1978 to 1979. In Foucault's *Security, Territory and Population* (2009), it is argued that governments no longer operate according to the old paradigm of governing bodies but according to the paradigm of governing entire populations. While Foucault's analyses were focused on the development of the biopolitical paradigm during the modern era, Agamben expanded this by tracing it to ancient Rome, specifically in Roman juridico-political texts where a specific class of human beings are relocated in a legal space which they may be sacrificed without contravening any legal prohibitions. This 'state of exception' continues in the left since it pervades in the time of democratic-revolutionary traditions in Western political thought (Agamben 2005: 5).

If we are to imagine that the revolutionary movements could save us from state power, nothing could be further from the truth. In the hands of Napoleon, the revolutionary *par excellence*, the Roman 'state of exception' is transformed into the concept of '*the state of siege*' in his decree of December 24, 1811, during the Revolutionary period. In this decree, it was held that the emperor could declare whether the city was in a 'state of war'. The significance of this is that when a city is declared to be in 'a state of war', police power will be transferred to the military. While this doctrine was initially conceived as a response to exceptional circumstances, so that they can defend military strongholds more effectively, with the declared aim of defending the population, one ironic consequence of this is that the population came to be seen as 'the enemy'. This occurred with the gradual emancipation of this doctrine from wartime situations to peaceful conditions, so that extraordinary police measures are now authorized *at all times* in the city to cope with 'internal sedition' and disorder. In such a 'state of exception', the executive branch of the sovereign gained 'full powers' (*pleins pouvoirs*) to issue decrees that have the force of law. Thus, despite the universal axioms of the revolutionary left, they did not, *they could not*, avoid the inevitable rise of biopower.

If we somehow imagined that biopower came to an end in modern liberal democracies, then we would be disappointed too. Agamben's second book on this subject entitled the *State of Exception* (2005) argues that the executive's 'full powers' did not diminish but underwent expansion during the two world wars, heralding a condition in which the state of exception has become the reigning paradigm for modern governments. The most salient example of this is, as Agamben pointed out, in the 'military order' issued by the president of the United States on November 12, 2001. This order seemingly authorizes the 'indefinite detention' of noncitizens who are suspected of involvement in terrorist activities in a trial by conducted 'military commissions'. While citizens of America may applaud this development, what they don't seem to realize is that it has also expanded the power of the attorney general, who is now invested with the power to 'take into custody' anyone suspected of activities that endangered 'the national security of the United States' by the USA Patriot Act issued on October 26, 2001. What was novel with this 'military order' is that it also erases any legal status the individual may have, thus producing a legally unnamable and unclassifiable being, a being who in the language of classical political theory can be killed without either infringing human or sacrificial laws. This means that the Taliban captured in Afghanistan do not even have the status of POWs as defined by the Geneva Convention; they do not even have the status of persons charged with the most heinous crime in American laws (Agamben 2005: 3).

One consequence when the exception has become the norm is that it creates a space called 'the camp' right at the heart of the city. When what was supposed to be nothing but a temporary suspension of the rule of law in an area is now given *permanent* status; what has occurred is none other than the fact that the exception has become a 'fact' (Agamben 1998: 169). This leads to a condition in which what was excluded in the camp is, according to the etymological sense of the term 'exception' (*ex-capere*), *taken outside* or other words 'included through its own exclusion' (Agamben 1998: 170). This camp inaugurates a new 'juridico-political paradigm' in which the norm becomes totally indistinguishable from the exception – where the exception, based on a decision, becomes the norm. Agamben states that 'the camp is the space of this absolute impossibility of deciding between fact and law, rule and application, exception and rule, which nevertheless incessantly decides between them' (Agamben 1998: 173). According to Agamben, the camp is the 'paradigm' of a political space that lies at the point at which politics becomes *biopolitics*, and where citizen becomes *homo sacer*. Thus, Agamben holds that asking how such atrocities could be committed against human beings misses the point and is 'hypocritical'; the real question to ask is how human beings could be so deprived of their rights that no act committed against them could be seen as a crime (Agamben 1998: 171; 2000: 41). If the essence of the camp consists in the appearance of a state of exception in space in which life and bare life enter into a threshold of indistinction, then the implication for this is that we must admit that we find ourselves in a camp every time such a structure is created (Agamben 1998: 174). When this camp is securely lodged within the city's interior, the camp can be seen as the new norm (*nomos*) of the modern (Agamben 1998: 174–175; 2000: 45).

Agamben maintains that when the exception becomes the norm what is undermined is none other than parliamentary democracy itself. This is because laws of this nature, which belong to exceptional circumstances of necessity or emergency, conflict with the fundamental principles, hierarchy, and regulation of democratic institutions. As legal thinkers may say, 'when what was merely a temporary power becomes a systematic and regular exercise, it can only lead to the "liquidation" of democracy' (Tingsten 1934: 333; Agamben 2005: 6–7). Thus, in many states, parliamentary democracies are only democracies in name when they maintain the doctrine of the state of exception. In other words, the theories that justify emergency in the name of defending the democratic constitutions in fact lead to its ruin. As reiterated by Agamben, Friedrich states that:

> There are no ultimate institutional safeguards available for insuring that emergency powers be used for the purpose of preserving the Constitution. Only the people's own determination to see them so used can make sure of that … All in all the quasi-dictatorial provisions of modern constitutional systems, be they martial rule, state of siege, or constitutional emergency powers, fail to conform to any exacting standard of effective limitations upon a temporary concentration of powers. Consequently, all these systems are liable to be transformed into totalitarian schemes if conditions become favourable to it.
>
> *(Agamben 2005: 8)*

Agamben states that the state of exception is now neither external nor internal to the juridical order, and there is a problem in defining it is precisely because there is a threshold, or a zone of indifference where inside and outside do not exclude each other but rather blur with each other. And to understand the state of exception, one must correctly determine its localization or illocalization (Agamben 2005: 23–24).

Agamben's critique of biopolitics shares some similarities with ideological analysis in the sense that it assumes that the masses are misled by ideology to believe that their interests are aligned with that of the ruling class. This makes them support the ruling class because they are unable to see that their interests are fundamentally at odds with those of the ruling class. If ideological analyses are right, then the political task would be a straightforward one, namely, to overthrow the existing ruling class and to replace it with a revolutionary one. This in turn requires that the masses be sufficiently educated to such an extent that they are free from their ideological blinders and come to see the class conflict that lies hidden in plain sight. While this appears to be straightforward enough, it does not seem to be workable in practice. As Deleuze and Guattari have observed, the masses do not seem to be interested in being educated,

> We see the most disadvantaged, the most excluded members of society invest with passion the system that oppresses them, and where they always find an interest in it, since it is here that they search for and measure it. Interest always comes after.
>
> *(Deleuze and Guattari 1977: 346)*

Hence, ideological analysts often find their own interests at odds with the very masses that they seek to liberate.

Deleuze and Guattari and the Politics of Desire

Deleuze and Guattari are known for criticizing ideological approaches because they focus on the conscious and ignore the unconscious. Deleuze and Guattari follow Nietzsche in assuming the primacy of the unconscious over the conscious. Deleuze and Guattari pointed out that much of human motivation does not result from rational calculations but occurs outside our conscious awareness. Human reason is, in a sense, as David Hume once pointed out, the slave of the passions. Deleuze once stated that

> Underneath the self which acts are little selves which contemplates and which render possible both the action and the active subject. We speak of our "self" only in virtue of these thousands of little witnesses which contemplate within us: it is always a third party who says "me".
>
> *(Deleuze & Guattari 1994: 75)*

In *Difference and Repetition* (1994), Deleuze calls such forms of thinking a 'dogmatic image of thought' – since they do not take into account difference but try to subsume difference under the Same and the Similar. Such thinking passes for thinking but in fact eliminates thinking under the image of the Same and the Similar. Ultimately, such a form of thinking serves practical, moral, and ultimately political forces that have fascist arrangements.

Specifically, Deleuze and Guattari criticize the ideological approach because it is obsessed with the cognitive aspect and neglects the affective-cognitive aspect of motivation. In other words, it neglects the fundamental starting point of motivation, and that is none other than desire. For Deleuze and Guattari, it is important to engage with the question of desire because it is in understanding desire that we can understand why people support fascist regimes:

> Reich is at his greatest as a thinker when he refuses to accept ignorance or illusion on the part of the masses as an explanation of fascism, and demands an explanation in terms of desire: no, the masses were not duped, under certain circumstances they desired fascism, and it is this perversion of mass desire we have to explain.
>
> *(Deleuze and Guattari 1977: 29–30)*

As Deleuze and Guattari would say, the critique of ideology got it from the wrong end when it seeks to correct the apparent irrationality that is at work in society by focusing on the powers that disseminate such illusions instead of focusing on the masses that support such powers. For Deleuze and Guattari, the real action is not in the political system but in understanding the perverse desires of the masses, desires that seek their own repression and ultimate destruction. Hence, they say that outward behaviour is:

> not a question of ideology. There is an unconscious libidinal investment of the social field, which coexists but does not necessarily coincide with preconscious investments, or with that which the preconscious investments "should be." That's why, when subjects – individuals or groups – go manifestly against their class interests, when they adhere to the interests and ideas of a class that their own objective situation should determine them to combat, it's not enough to say: they have been fooled, the masses have been fooled. It's not an ideological problem of misrecognition and illusion, it's a problem of desire, *and desire is part of the infrastructure.*
>
> *(1977: 104)*

For Deleuze and Guattari, one of the central themes of *Anti-Oedipus* is that *desire is productive*. What this means is that *desire directly creates its objects*. In a similar vein, it is desire that produces the social. Of course, desire may create fascist arrangements that in turn repress or distort desire, but this does not displace the primacy of desire in production. In a sense, desire and the social are not distinct and separate from each other. Desiring-production is the direct libidinal investment in how the structure operates. So in a major study on Deleuze and Guattari's engagement with fascism by Evans and Reid (2013), it is simply not true that fascist ideologues somehow managed to mislead the masses; rather it is the masses that desire fascist arrangements in the first place, which led to the rise of fascist ideologues. Thus, in Deleuze and Guattari's analysis, fascism is not simply a political ideology perpetrated by an elite upon an unwitting and subdued masses, but the very expression of the desire of the masses itself; it is an unconscious 'desiring machine' that is able to mobilize the conscious desire of a people for its own repression.

This explains why Deleuze and Guattari demonstrated an almost complete lack of interest in much of the political commitments and debates that characterize Anglo-American thought. Deleuze and Guattari's analysis does not engage in such debates because it is not a question of which political system is superior but what are the drives of the masses to support those systems. Likewise, Deleuze and Guattari seem less interested in the question of fascism than in the question of what gave rise to fascist regimes in the first place. This brings to mind Foucault's 'Preface' to Deleuze and Guattari's *Anti-Oedipus* project when he states that

> the major enemy, the strategic adversary is fascism ... and not only historical fascism, the fascism of Hitler and Mussolini ... but also the fascism in us all, in our heads and our everyday behaviour, the fascism that causes us to love power, to desire the very thing that dominates and exploits us.
>
> *(Deleuze and Guattari 1977: xiii)*

So Deleuze and Guattari's analyses redirect our attention from fascist systems to the drives and desires that support those systems.

This explains why Deleuze and Guattari did not support democratic systems simply because they are democratic. This is because they are all equally capable of becoming despotic. In fact, as Deleuze and Guattari might say, many democratic states are already compromised and are complicit in their role in the production of human misery alongside great wealth that is produced by the globalized system of exploitation (Deleuze and Guattari 1994: 107). To be sure, their lack of support for democratic norms does not mean that they support non-democratic or even anti-democratic systems such as authoritarian or even fascist ones. Deleuze and Guattari are known for supporting utopic political visions that are immanent, revolutionary, and libertarian. They give priority to minoritarian becomings rather than majoritarian beings, to planes of consistency rather than planes of organization, to nomadic machines rather than apparatuses of capture. In doing so, Deleuze and Guattari follow Nietzsche in seeing politics not in terms of static arrangements. The state form appeared in human history in the guise of different kinds of despotic machines. When one state replaces another, it is just one despotic machine replacing another despotic machine. Therefore, there is no point in debating as to which arrangement is superior to others because so long as it exists in the form of the state, its despotic potential is there.

The Schizoanalysis and Deterrritorialization of Biopolitics

If Deleuze and Guattari considered ideological critiques to be wrong headed, they regarded philosophy in terms of schizoanalysis and deterritorialization to be critical. Deleuze maintained in an interview with Negri that 'Anti-Oedipus was from the beginning to end a work of political philosophy' (Deleuze & Guattari 1994: 170) without affirming any political system to be the cure for all. Hence, it has been controversial whether Deleuze offered any political ideas at all. We get a hint in *What Is Philosophy?* (1994), when Deleuze and Guattari follow Nietzsche in defining philosophy as an activity which involves the creation of concepts that are 'untimely' because it involves a critique of the time in which one lives. Secondly, they reserve the 'utopian' function of philosophy in the sense of summoning 'a new earth and a people that does not yet exist' (Deleuze and Guattari 1994: 108).

The first task of philosophy, what they have come to call "schizoanalysis," then, is none other than to recognize the libidinal investments in fascist formations and then to see how we can make those investments more revolutionary. Deleuze and Guattari state this quite clearly when they say that 'The first positive task consists in discovering in a subject the nature, the formation, or functioning of his desiring-machines, independent of any interpretations' (Deleuze and Guattari 1977: 322). The second task of philosophy is none other than 'deterritorialization'. This concept can be found *Anti-Oedipus* (1977), and it is further expanded in *A Thousand Plateaus* (1987). It is finally applied to the question of thinking in *What Is Philosophy?* (1994). Through the concept of deterritorialisation Deleuze and Guattari make a distinction between 'earth' and 'territory'. Territory refers to eterritorializ earth that has its own movements of eterritorialization, and the earth also contains processes of eterritorialization and the constitution of new territories. Stable identities or territories are therefore secondary formations upon the mobile earth. This philosophy is utopian in the sense that it constantly opens up the possibility of new forms of individual and collective identity, thereby effecting the absolute eterritorialization of the present in thought.

In the context of the current crisis, I believe it is legitimate to ask whether a schizoanalysis of biopolitics is possible. While Agamben's insights into the rise of biopolitics is no doubt valuable, we must also ask what are the unconscious desires that lead to the rise of such a form of politics. That is, instead of being overly obsessed with the correct political system, we should turn our attention to what is the desire that led to the rise of the biopolitical paradigm. What are the libidinal investments that the masses have poured into the rise of biopolitics? Why do people quietly accept state paradigms that view them as 'population' and 'statistics' instead of viewing them as citizens with rights? Why do believe with all their heart and all their might that surveillance technologies and movement controls are the way to go? Why do people focus exclusively on vaccines as the solution to the coronavirus instead of other options? What have the vaccines got to do with the medical industry and capitalism? I believe that by turning our attention to the unconscious desire of the masses, it would make Agamben's analysis of biopolitics more meaningful.

Furthermore, I believe it is also important to ask whether in what ways the rise of biopolitics in the wake of the coronavirus has deterritorialised existing territories. I believe that the coronavirus for the first time in human history impresses upon us the inability of traditional national boundaries to deliver the promised security. The high infection rates and death rates, when combined with new mutant forms of the virus with its ability to spread across the globe in a matter of days, renders obsolete the territorial delimitations of traditional concepts of sovereignty. Its effectiveness also points to the end of the traditional military industrial complex that has besieged humanity for decades. This means that we can no longer rest on our traditional understanding of politics which is based on territory, borders, and discipline and have to start thinking of how we may have to move to a politics based on mutual responsibility. In such a condition, instead of a permanent individualized fear, which can break down any sense of social cohesion, we move to the idea of collective effort, coordination, and solidarity within a common struggle, elements that in such health emergencies can be equally important to medical interventions. This can also be based on the democratisation of knowledge. The increased access to knowledge, along with the need for popularisation campaigns, makes possible collective decision processes that are based on knowledge and understanding and not just the authority of transcendent experts. Agamben's philosophy analysed the switch from *zoe* to *bios* in Western political thought, but the coronavirus has opened up an occasion for a return to politics of life as *zoe*. In other words, we have to start asking ourselves whether we have had enough of biopolitics and whether there is still time to desire a *zoepolitics*.

Bibliography

Agamben, Giorgio. 1998. *Homo Sacer: Sovereign Power and Bare Life*. Translated by Daniel Heller-Roazen. Stanford & California: Stanford University Press.

Agamben, Giorgio. 2000. *Potentialities: Collected Essays in Philosophy*. Translated by Daniel Heller-Roazen. Stanford: Stanford University Press.

Agamben, Giorgio. 2003. *The Coming Community*. Translated by Michael Hardt. Minneapolis: University of Minnesota Press.

Agamben, Giorgio. 2005. *State of Exception*. Translated by Kevin Attell. Chicago & London: University of Chicago Press.

Agamben, Giorgio. 2020. *Means without Ends: Notes on Politics*. Translated by Vincenzo Binetti and Cesare Casarino. London and Minneapolis: University of Minnesota Press.

Agamben, Giorgio. 2020. *The Invention of an Epidemic* (Italian), *Quodlibet*, https://www.quodlibet.it/giorgio-agamben-l-invenzione-di-un-epidemia)

Agamben, Giorgio. 2021. *Where Are We Now? The Epidemic as Politics*. Translated by V. Dani. Lanham, MA: Rowman and Littlefield.

Buchanan, Ian. 2008. *Deleuze and Guattari's Anti-Oedipus*. London: Continuum.

Deleuze, Gilles and Felix Guattari. 1977. *Anti-Oedipus: Capitalism and Schizophrenia*. New York: Viking Press.

Deleuze, Gilles and Felix Guattari. (1994). *What Is Philosophy?* Translated by H. TomlInson and G. Burchell. New York: Columbia University Press.

Deleuze, Gilles and Felix Guattari. 2003. *Anti-Oedipus: Capitalism & Schizophrenia*. London: Athlone Press.

Deleuze, Gilles and Felix Guattari. 2012. *Anti-Oedipus*. Translated by Robert Hurley, Mark Seem and Helen R. Lane. London and New York: Continuum.

Evans, Brad and Julian Reid (eds.). 2013. *Deleuze & Fascism Security: War: Aesthetics*. London, New York: Routledge.

Foucault, Michel. 1977/2008. 'Preface' in Gilles Deleuze and Felix Guattari (eds), *Anti-Oedipus: Capitalism & Schizophrenia*. London: Athlone Press.

Foucault, Michel. 2009. *Security, Territory, Population: Lectures at the College De France 1977–1978*, Michel Senelart (ed.), Translated by Graham Burchell, London: Palgrave.

Foucault, Michel. n.d. *The Birth of Biopolitics: Lectures at the College De France 1978–1979*, Michel Senelart (ed.), Translated by Graham Burchell. London: Palgrave.

Guattari, Felix. 2006. *The Anti-Oedipus Papers*, Stephane Nadaud (ed.), Translated by Kelina Gotman. New York: Semiotext(e).

Patton, Paul. 2000. *Deleuze and the Political*. London and New York: Routledge.

Tingsten, Herbert. 1934. *Les pleins pouvoirs: l'expansion des pouvoirs gouvernementaux pendant et après la grande guerre*. Paris: Librairie Stock.

8

OF VIRUS AND MAN

From Wound to Belief in the World

Sebastian Hsien-Hao Liao

The Birth of the Paranoiac

In the epochal disruption caused by the viral event of the Covid-19 pandemic, governments and specialists scrambled to cope with this almost apocalyptic situation. Unfortunately, as Bishop and Fitzgerald observe, most of the responses have been products of some form of humanist cosmopolitanism which simply are not able to consider the big picture where the virus has become the agent-protagonist (2020: 1). But actually, in order to have a broader vision, one that could take in all aspects of this event, we don't really have to look far. What is needed is but a currently much discussed posthumanist approach that can redress the humanist blindness toward the human's inextricably interrelated but neglected companion – the nonhuman world. And the most appropriate place to begin is no doubt a re-think of the human–virus relationship, which this pandemic conveniently has enabled.

As a matter of fact, contemplation on the virus has not been rare in the last few decades. And one can even go so far to say that the virus has been used as a master trope for the postmodern condition (Bardini 2011: 179). Powerful thinkers such as William Burroughs, Baudrillard, Derrida, and Deleuze have quite productively reflected on the phenomenon of virus. It is, however, interesting to note that this trope has been used in both directions. On the one hand, Burroughs, Baudrillard, and Derrida warned that we have been infected by viruses of one kind or another of which the symptoms have run amok, while on the other, the trope of virus has also been deployed both by Derrida and Deleuze as the very weapon to fight what they believe to be the major

DOI: 10.4324/9781003507789-10

illness of our time. And Deleuze (and Guattari) even developed a viral ontology that treats the virus pharmacologically.

In other words, the trope of virus is at once the human illness and the antidote to that same illness. Understood as illness, the trope refers to what has infected postmodern culture at its core (Bardini 2011: 189). But what exactly this illness is has been variously identified. William Burroughs sees words (and images) as viruses that create hybridized human beings but also limit the hybridizing by means of control (Land 2005: 453–457). Baudrillard considers terrorism as a virus, which has become a suicidal banality in the postmodern capitalist system (Baudrillard 2003: 1–35). With Derrida, we began to approach a viral ontology. Derrida has identified the illness as "autoimmunity" of which terrorism is one of its major symptoms (Bardini 2011: 187–188). But Esposito has defined this illness in clearer terms when he identified it as the immunological nature of modern politics. The impulse of modern communities to "protect" their purity by defending against viral contamination from unneeded elements generates immuno-political paranoia. Eventually, it turns into the problem of autoimmunity precisely because of the reversal caused by the obsession to immunize against the viral elements (Neyrat 2010: 32–34). But it is Deleuze and Guattari who truly see the pharmacological nature of the virus both as is and as a trope.[1] That is, for them it is from the same virus that has been devastating the humans since time immemorial that we hope to extract the antidotes to it.

Even though disease-causing viruses, along with other pathogens, have been the nemesis to the human beings ever since the latter climbed down the trees and started territorializing the earth, turning it increasingly into human habitats (McNeill), viruses benign to the human beings are also legion. The human genome, for instance, is even at least 45 percent composed of sequences related to retroviruses, not to mention viruses' other beneficial contributions to human health and growth (Moelling & Broecker 2019: 7–8). And the kind of viral ontology that Deleuze and Guattari proffer has been modeled on precisely the existing but little understood human–nonhuman relationship, one that Deleuze and Guattari describe as "aparallel" evolution where the human and the virus, for example, mutually penetrate and co-mingle:

> [There is no] imitation at all but a capture of code, surplus value of code, an increase in valence, a veritable becoming, a becoming-wasp of the orchid and a becoming-orchid of the wasp. Each of these becomings brings about the deterritorialization of one term and the reterritorialization of the other; the two becomings interlink and form relays in a circulation of intensities pushing the deterritorialization ever further. There is neither imitation nor resemblance, only an exploding of two heterogeneous series on the line of flight composed by a common rhizome that can no longer be attributed to or subjugated by anything signifying. Rémy Chauvin

> expresses it well: "The aparallel evolution of two beings that have absolutely nothing to do with each other."
>
> *(Deleuze and Guattari 1987: 10)*

While the nonhuman world is both beneficial and inimical to the human being, this kind of evolution, also called symbiosis, is the rule rather than exception to how "nature" evolves.

But ever since the human beings began to expand their territory, the struggle between the human and nonhuman has become increasingly intense, and viruses detrimental to human health, along with other pathogens, have occupied a disproportionate amount of our attention. Modernity especially is obsessed with "controlling" the risks posed by the nonhuman world. And that ironically has provoked even more violent revenge from the nonhuman, which is manifested among other things in plagues (Mythen and Beck 2004).

Before we proceed to delve further into the Deleuzian viral ontology for a better understanding of what we are facing in this pandemic and how we are to cope with it, let's first investigate why there is the human impulse to control what we consider to be the heterogeneous elements or risk. For this, Deleuze and Guattari's *Anti-Oedipus* (2009) has a thorough discussion which unfolds as a critique of Freudian psychoanalysis. It is the Oedipus, they argue, that produces this almost universal paranoiac tendency in the modern man. But it is not Oedipus as a universal rule that creates the capitalist machine, but the other way round: "we have never dreamed of saying that psychoanalysis invented Oedipus. Everything points in the opposite direction: the subjects of psychoanalysis arrive already oedipalized" (Deleuze and Guattari 2009: 121). The deciding moment was when capitalism transformed the family structure into the bourgeois nuclear family romance of "father–mother–the child" to accommodate the capitalist system of "capital–earth–worker" (Deleuze and Guattari 2009: 264). As Deleuze and Guattari argue,

> In short, Oedipus arrives: it is born in the capitalist system of the application of first-order social images to the private familial images of the second order. It is the aggregate of destination that corresponds to an aggregate of departure that is socially determined. It is our intimate colonial formation that corresponds to the form of social sovereignty. We are all little colonies and it is Oedipus that colonizes us.
>
> *(Deleuze and Guattari 2009: 65)*

In short, concludes Eugene Holland, "the nuclear family as a specifically capitalist institution internalizes and then reproduces the Oedipal social dynamic of the capitalist market" (2002: 29).

The bourgeois nuclear family that emerged with the capitalist modernity has trained desire to invest in the "Oedipal territoriality", one that coheres closely with capitalism which intensely engages in privatizing reproduction and production as well as distinguishing them, and thereby domesticates desire (Holland 2002: 27–28). It is by means of repressing the desiring machine that the capitalist system makes an Oedipal/capitalist subject:

> the paranoiac investment consists in subordinating molecular desiring-production to the molar aggregate it forms on one surface of the full body without organs, enslaving it by that very fact to a form of socius that exercises the function of a full body under determinate conditions.
>
> *(Deleuze and Guattari 2009: 364)*

This subordination of desiring production, alternately called "productive unconscious", is instrumental in turning us into paranoiacs. For, argues Lapoujade (2014: 191), "The limit must preserve an identity of unalloyed purity, protect its territorialities from foreign infiltrations or invisible spies; it must shield a healthy body from microbes and filth. The paranoid is the guardian of limits". That is why Deleuze and Guattari (2009: 278) observe that "Oedipus is a dependency of the paranoiac territoriality", and thus anyone born in an Oedipal milieu is trained to be paranoiac. In other words, it is the Oedipus that has turned us all into paranoiacs who are consistently prone to control. And the extensive stratifying in all aspects of human existence as a result of paranoia has prompted Deleuze and Guattari to promote schizoid moves to counter the former. Fleeing from the ubiquitous and perennial Urstaat, schizoid moves are "lines of escape" that are "singularly creative and positive" (Deleuze and Guattari 2009: 376). Being the "two poles of unconscious libidinal investment", the paranoiac and the schizoid work in opposing directions. The paranoiac investment

> subordinates desiring-production to the formation of sovereignty and to the gregarious aggregate that results from it, while the other [the schizoid] brings about the inverse subordination, overthrows the established power, and subjects the gregarious aggregate to the molecular multiplicities of the productions of desire.
>
> *(Deleuze and Guattari 2009: 376)*

In other words, the schizoid investment initiates rhizomatic flights with a view toward breaking through paranoiac territorialization and benefiting from an experience of blurring the boundaries between self and the world (Deleuze and Guattari 2009: 9).

The Event as Wound

Hence, the importance of the event. For the event is what can precipitate schizoid or rhizomatic flights. The Deleuzian notion of "event" is basically derived from the fundamental distinction made by the Stoics between two realms of being, a material realm of bodies and states of affairs and an incorporeal realm of events. Thus, the event is on the one hand grounded in the body and on the other incorporeal and impersonal (Patton 1997: 2; Sellars 2006: 160). The point about these two different understandings of the event is that they make clear the two opposing processes enabled by the event: the counter-actualization (counter-effectuation) caused by the event and the actualization (effectuation) of the event (Deleuze 2003: 151). On the double structure of the event, Deleuze has further elaborated as follows:

> With every event, there is indeed the present moment of its actualization, the moment in which the event is embodied in a state of affairs, an individual, or a person, the moment we designate by saying 'here, the moment has come.' The future and the past of the event are evaluated only with respect to this definitive present, and from the point of view of that which embodies it. But on the other hand, there is the future and the past of the event considered in itself, sidestepping each present, being free of the limitations of a state of affairs, impersonal and pre-individual, neutral, neither general nor particular, eventum tantum. ... It has no other present than that of the mobile instant which represents it, always divided into past-future, and forming what must be called the counter-actualization.
>
> *(Deleuze 2003: 151)*

Actualization pertains to the event in historical time (Chronos) while counter-actualization pertains to the pure event of unlimited cosmic time (Aion) (Deleuze 2003: 53–61; Patton 1997: 8). Even as the event takes place in historical time, the pure event, by means of the procedure of counter-actualization, ushers the patient thinker[2] into the time of Aion where the patient thinker is able to access the plane of immanence or the Event. While Chronos provides the event with a description (representation), Aion endows the patient thinker with a perspective of cosmic time where the present melts into both the future and the past. But the pure event always subsists and insists in the actualized event (Deleuze 2003: 53; Sellars 2006: 164).

The Covid-19 pandemic is certainly one of the most salient events human beings have ever encountered and which no Deleuzian would fail to so construe. While being a most extreme heterogeneous element that flouts human control, the pandemic as event is in the same breath immensely beneficial, being able to provide rhizomatic flights from the mechanisms of control. In other words, the pandemic and for that matter all events can be construed pharmacologically both as scourge and cure, which coincidentally echoes the myth of Pandora's Box which both releases plagues among other things and retains hope.

While it may have been banal by now to discuss the evental implications of this pandemic, I believe its potential as event has not been exhausted. I would like to call attention to the concomitant notion of "wound" in order to deepen our understanding of the event in general and this pandemic in particular and of how we can cope with the latter in a radical manner. That is, only by combining the concept of "wound" with the event can we realize how events have the power to counter-actualize, throwing us into the time of Aion for accessing the plane of immanence.

The wound is not this or that actual wound we as individuals sustain in everyday life, but an existential or virtual situation (Williams 2008: 12). Like the event, there are also two dimensions of the wound, the actual and the incorporeal. What this means is that while in actuality a wound may be physical or emotional, the incorporeal wound reveals a fundamental 'crack' in the human being's existence which is silently creeping and expanding until the right moment arrives for it to turn into an actualized crack (Deleuze 2003: 155–157). The incorporeal wound is immanence or the virtual which contains the eternal truth (Deleuze 2003: 53, 64; Deleuze 1997a: 31–32). But only with the articulation of these two cracks can the fundamental truth of the incorporeal wound be revealed.

But before we proceed to discuss how these two wounds can be articulated, a further question must be asked: Where then does the incorporeal wound originate? In *Logic of Sense*, Deleuze (2003) basically argues from a psychoanalytical perspective and refers this wound to the constitutive split of the human subjectivity by language. The crack on the surface of the subject/patient-thinker is created by language's incision in the impersonal and the pre-individual which fractures the subject into a body that struggles to express on the one hand and the language system that presumably speaks on behalf of the body on the other. In fact, Deleuze (2003: 208) explicitly indicates that the crack corresponds to the "trace of castration" or "narcissistic wound", and later on also manifests itself in the "double direction" of events which "fragments the subject". The "entire sexual surface", with castration as the core, serves as the "intermediary between physical depth and metaphysical surface" (Deleuze 2003: 222). That is also why Deleuze observes most cryptically that sexuality and thought are connected (Deleuze 2003: 219): for it is quite clear to Deleuze that what psychoanalysis is talking about by pivoting to castration is events and the wound (Deleuze 2003: 211). And Joe Bousquet's remark that Deleuze consistently quotes validates this reading: "my wound existed before me, I was born to embody it" (Deleuze 2003: 148). The physical wound that incapacitated him reveals an existential wound that predates his consciousness. What else but the entry into language or consciousness inflicts this wound?[3]

Sense Is Nonsense

Thus, the first wound (trauma) is the fundamental human wound, which is inflicted on the human subject at the moment of entering into the world of language and termed the "wound of castration" or "crack constitutive of thought" (Deleuze 2003: 219). All later wounds (events) in actuality would have to connect with this wound to make real sense. For only when counter-actualization occurs can thought "take the chance to imagine things differently" (Williams 2008: 192). But thought has an ambiguous relationship with language. And to elaborate on this relationship, in *Logic of Sense*, Deleuze has carefully distinguished three stages of the dynamic genesis of language: "(1) the primary order is the noise produced in the depths of the body; (2) the secondary organization constitutes the surface of sense (and non-sense); and (3) the tertiary arrangement [ordonnance] is found in fully-formed propositions, with their functions of denotation, manifestation, and signification" (Smith and Protevi 2020). The first sees the infant still caught in their body, acting purely on instincts. In the second stage, the infant learns how to organize noises into sense. But sense here is intertwined with non-sense, or more accurately, alternates between sense and nonsense, operating mainly on "esoteric words". In the third stage, the child has managed to use language in all its functions (Deleuze 2003: 239–249).

But the important thing is that, with the three stages becoming later in life three different orders of language/being, Deleuze actually values the second stage above the third. For the third is already the language of the State whereas the second with its potential of 'nonsense' is able to disrupt the language of the State with events and force us to think.[4] And sense in fact, observes Williams, "must be associated with his concept of the virtual as developed in *Difference and Repetition*" where "sense corresponds to the multiplicity of virtual Ideas and to the intensities that are expressed in virtual Ideas and in their actualisations" (2008: 31). Having an in-between status, sense is that which enables language (propositions) on the one hand and what counter-actualization consistently returns to on the other:

> Sense is both the expressible or the expressed of the proposition, and the attribute of the state of affairs. It turns one side toward things, and another side toward propositions. But it cannot be confused with the proposition which expressed it any more than with the state of affairs or the quality which the proposition denotes. It is exactly the boundary between propositions and things.
>
> *(Deleuze 2003: 22)*

In other words, sense is the plane of immanence, neither complete chaos nor transcendence constructed by the representational tendency in language.

Thus, language is double-edged. On the one hand, it is transcendent-prone, but on the other it contains a foreign tongue in it, that is, sense which, being nonsense from the point of view of the language system, contains the seeds of renewal and creativity – events (Deleuze 2003: 211; Williams 2008: 72).[5]

So how are we going to face up to an event and the wound it is definitely going to inflict upon us? The important thing is to actively "search for the eternal side of our wounds" (Williams 2008: 151). And it is by means of connecting the two dimensions of the wound, the actual and the incorporeal, that the patient thinker can be enabled to see the full range of possibilities on the plane of immanence. But since not everyone is fit for evental encounters (Zourabichvili 1994: 91), the crack or wound is often papered over by the language system and conveniently serves as an easy stepping stone to a transcendent world view. Thus, there needs to be a more proactive approach to ensure the connection of the two dimensions, given that the wound would not let go anyway as "there is necessarily a flaw in all things because they matter – because they have a sense" (Williams 2008: 160). What is advisable for us to do is follow steadfastly the advice of the Stoics to "become worthy of what happens to us" and "will and release the event" (Deleuze 2003: 149). But this proactive approach ironically presupposes that one can adopt the principle of apparently passive attitude of "amor fati" in the face of the wound (Deleuze 2003: 151).

What Nietzsche means by amor fati is to accept the result of any throw of dice but try in the same breath to make the best of it. And this attempt presupposes the ability to counter-actualize so as to avail oneself of all the virtual possibilities before deciding what best to do. Thus, despite seeming like a passive acceptance of fate, it in fact involves a creative act that tries to find the best option for the current situation. And above all, this attempt requires a reformulation of the problem itself. That is why, following Bergson, Deleuze argues that

> [t]rue freedom lies in a power to decide, to constitute problems themselves. For Bergson, this freedom is even considered semi-divine ..., probably the only power that can be considered freedom. And this "semi-divine" power entails the disappearance of false problems as much as the creative upsurge of true ones.
>
> *(Deleuze 1988a: 15)*

Somewhat differently put, the "greatest freedom" is "the freedom by which we develop and lead the event to its completion" (Deleuze 2003: 212). And the whole point about Deleuze's philosophy is probably how to attain this freedom. And paradoxically it can be attained only through amor fati.

To exemplify (the failure to attain) this freedom, Deleuze cites the example of the Chinese professor Yu Tsun in Borges' immensely famous short story "The Garden of Forking Paths". Yu Tsun, formerly a professor of English in the Chinese city Tsingtao, has been forced into working as a secret agent for the Germans who had seized Tsingtao as their colony. Yu Tsun's task is to locate the site of an artillery park and transmit the name thereof to the chief of intelligence in Berlin whom he actually detests. When Yu figures out that he can pass this message onto his boss by killing a British sinologist who is coincidentally an expert on his grandfather's philosophy of time, he is somehow in a quandary. With only one bullet left in his revolver and the agent from the British intelligence closing in on him, what should he do? To kill or not to kill? The high point of this whole event is when Yu Tsun is rendered aware of the philosophy of time proposed by his grandfather, a philosophy that presents time as constantly forking and makes available to him all the virtual possibilities in handling the current situation. But eventually Yu does not reformulate his problem; he is still caught in the old problem of "how to pass the intelligence on to his German boss" rather than formulate it into a new one such as "how should I best deal with this situation where in fact I have multiple choices rather than only two".

For someone like Yu Tsun who is an example of a deeply colonized subject, paranoia has become a habit insofar as he is always trying to win recognition from the colonial authorities so as to fill up the gaping lack/crack in his subjectivity. As a result, he is not able to become a body without organs and to actually adopt other alternatives. For him, the plane of immanence is but an ephemeral glimpse where for a short instant he feels the swarming of all alternatives. As mentioned earlier, not everyone is fit for this kind of encounter (Zourabichvili 1994: 91), for events are "problematic and problematizing" (Deleuze 2003: 54). And thus some people prefer the tree rather than the rhizome.

The Object's Wound

The foregoing discussion about how to cope with the wound inflicted by an event may nevertheless seem like an anthropocentric project. But it is only half the story, for the nonhuman world is also composed of agents and therefore has its side of the story to tell, too. When Deleuze and Guattari observe that we ought to "give birth to new modes of existence, closer to animals and rocks" (Deleuze and Guattari 1994: 74–75), they are obviously suggesting that in adjusting our modes of existence, we emulate those of animals and rocks. This implies that, for Deleuze and Guattari, the animals and rocks have superior modes of existence. But in what way does this proclamation stand? In light of the spirit of Deleuzian ontology, one would be tempted to say that they do not use languages and therefore live an immanent mode of existence.

But to be more precise, the reason should be ascribed to the fact that animals and rocks do not use human languages. Even though they seem apparently language-less, they may have other kinds of "languages". In fact, Deleuze himself uses the example of a "cleft rock" to give expression to the fact that even a rock has its own way of dealing with its crack (Deleuze 2003: 155–156). And, to coordinate human and nonhuman ways of making sense, James Williams explains that the porcelain in the title to the 22nd series in *Logic of Sense*

> is an allusion to the belief that any actual thing is necessarily flawed under its actual surface because its significance and value put it in touch with paradoxes and tensions that belie any claim to perfection. Put simply, there is necessarily a flaw in all things because they matter – because they have a sense.
>
> *(Williams 2008: 160)*

The fact that any object can be using some kind of language pertaining to it can be further understood with OOO's description of how an object always has a crack within. Though not having to undergo a process of Oedipality, the object is also born to be split by their having to enter into relations with the external world. In other words, where there is a relation, there is translation. And that means in establishing a relationship there is always some kind of "language" involved. Objects are no exceptions. According to the OOO, there is a split between the part of the object that establishes contact with the external world and the part that is withdrawn from any contact, one that is reminiscent of the psychoanalytical construal of the human subject's split between the subject of enunciation and the subject of statement.[6] It follows that all the consequences of using languages could be identified in objects as well. With the split being the wound, some degree of paranoia and tendency to control, both being attempts to cover up the wound, must also characterize their mode of existence. And Timothy Morton actually construes the object's "ego" history as the record of its quasi-paranoiac attempts to heal the wound (2013: 198).

But if, according to Deleuze and Guattari, animals and rocks are more congenial to the plane of immanence than humans, that means their way of dealing with the wound must be somewhat different from that of the humans. Although their paranoia is also derived from the "death drive" inherent in the object's existence, the kinds of language they use are, however, closer to immanence than the human language. And that makes all the difference. In other words, their language tends to be based on force (the "movements and intensities") or Whitehead's "prehension" (1978: 75).[7] Having the language of force or "prehension" mitigates the need to construct a transcendent plane where one is always engaged in "moral" struggles as to whether or not an ideology is "good sense". Presumably this language enables the animals and rocks to engage only in affecting and being affected. Suffice it to say that this language communicates much better than the human language because it is the language of the body or more precisely the body without organs.

In other words, being closer to the plane of immanence indicates that the superiority of the modes of existence "closer animals and rocks" lies in the fact that "matter is immanently creative" (Deleuze and Guattari 1987: 343). Thus, always already accepting their fate (that is, not having an abstract system that leans toward the transcendent), they tend to reformulate the problem in their own way whenever necessary (though not necessarily able to have a "better" solution in the eyes of the human). And this always involves "reaching out" to the one that gets into relation with them by means of prehension (that is, affecting and being affected), for they are always already "body without organs". And thus the way they handle the wound would be much closer to the ideal of amor fati which I would argue is fundamental to a viral ontology.

The Viral Ontology

There is ample reason for such an ontology as having been inflected by amor fati to be named viral ontology. For among all objects the virus provides the most picturesque manifestation of the modality of affecting and being affected. And the way they constantly mutate lends full evidence to their fundamental attitude of amor fati in that they consistently reformulate their problems under different circumstances. More importantly, it forms a "block of becoming" that fits most conveniently with Deleuze and Guattari's definition of becoming in the sense that what results from a becoming that happens between the human and the virus is the block of becoming rather than a "human-virus" that descends from it (Deleuze and Guattari 1987: 238–239). And the virus exemplifies to us how this block of becoming actually works. It is this that we must learn from the virus: return to aparallel evolution which is true Deleuzian becoming. To do so, we must return to our body; not body as organism, but as "organism unbound" (Ansell-Pearson 1997: 120) or "body without organs". Only when we can manage to become body without organs can we actually form blocks of becoming.

Thus, what must be reckoned is that the kind of human–virus relationship is actually typical of human–nonhuman relationship. When epidemics and plagues caused by viruses as well as other pathogens impact us as events, we must adopt the principle of amor fati in order to counter-actualize and thereby see the full range of possibilities on the plane of immanence. Amor fati allows us to look our incorporeal wound in the eye and realize that we are never complete and insular subjects and always live symbiotically with other creatures and objects. This pandemic serves as a timely reminder and warning of human transgressions of the boundaries that should not have been transgressed. We must therefore feel thankful toward the virus and for that matter the whole nonhuman world. It is therefore crucial that we hold back our tendency to control and respect the nonhuman world while enjoying living creatively with it (1995: 176), a mode of symbiosis typified by "aparallel evolution".

But here learning from the virus means Deleuzian "becoming virus", which is neither "imitative" nor "structural" but "cosmic": For Deleuze and Guattari, "becoming everybody/everything ... brings into play the cosmos with its molecular components. Becoming everybody/everything (tout le monde) is to world (faire monde), to make a world (faire un monde)" (Deleuze and Guattari 1987: 280). What results from this "learning", then, is not knowledge but faith derived from a cosmic communication across what Deleuze calls "positive distance" (Deleuze 2003: 172–173),[8] given that all events participate in the Event as the virtual and therein events communicate with each other (Deleuze 2003: 53, 64, 175–176). Thus, James Williams concludes that "we are eternally connected but provisionally separate" (2008: 167) with a very illuminating exegesis of Deleuze's notion of communication of all events in the Event:

> In short, when we express infinitives such as 'to love' or 'to hate' we must do so through what is different in our singular expression because the infinitive itself is only difference or a potential to be expressed differently and to connect differently to other infinitives. So any togetherness is not one that suffers and fails through the infinity of actual identifiable differences, but one that connects because it resists identity and is the genetic condition for the production of novel differences. It is because the infinitive can be expressed differently that we connect through the multiple ways we express it. When we do so we change the distances between infinitives and affirm their connection across those differences. This is no longer a world where there can be absolute oppositions or perfect identities. It is one where we are necessarily part of a community because the reality we express is one of communication through divergences, through disjunctive syntheses.
>
> *(Williams 2008: 167)*

This ability to live and let live is, however, not commonly found in a modern man, given that, according to Deleuze, we have lost the world. It then requires a more profound move to reclaim this ability: a commitment to regaining "belief in the world" on which the call to co-exist is premised. Deleuze (and Guattari) has consistently lamented the loss of belief in the world in his oeuvre and emphatically indicated that this is the most urgent problem of our times (Deleuze and Guattari 1994: 75; Deleuze 1989: 171–172; Deleuze 1995b: 176). By "believing in the world", however, he is not talking about whether or not to believe in the existence of the world but "the world, as it is" (Deleuze 1989: 172). This "as it is" has created similar misunderstandings as has the notion of amor fati or "becoming worthy of the event": that this is "an expression of resignation or ultimate acceptance of the limits that determine the world" (Thiele 2010: 35). But the fact is that the addition of "as it is", continues Kathrin Thiele, indicates "the paradoxical formulation of the only movement that might lead to real transformation: active affirmation of 'what is' in order to become inscribed in a dynamic process and thus re-acquire the potential to create something new" (2010: 35). In other words, "the world, as it is" is the world always already in the process of becoming. What Deleuze and Guattari are concerned about is reclaim the becoming "immanence ... immanent only to itself" (Deleuze and Guattari 1994: 45). And what the event does is precisely to transfer us to a "different plane" which is the plane of immanence where we can "give birth to new modes of existence, closer to animals and rocks" (Deleuze and Guattari 1994: 74–75).

Having a mode of existence much closer to animals and rocks than the humans, the coronavirus seemingly coming out of nowhere actually emerged from the depth of the Anthropocene. It is a sign, an esoteric word, a phantasm, that beckons us to "believe in the world" again by eluding control from anthropocentrism, among other things. And this imperative can be carried out by means of engaging in a becoming that involves the human being and the virus through which the two parties communicate with each other as well as with everything else in the Event (Zourabichvili 1994: 39; Williams 2008: 167), a Stoic cosmic becoming or the Tao where "the boundary between the individual and Nature is overcome, and there is no longer an opposition between the will of the individual and the will of God, which is identified with fate" (Sellars 2006: 164).

Notes

1 Even though Derrida also developed an incipient argument along the same lines as that of Deleuze, that is, introducing the virus into the I (Brunette and Wills 12), he failed to turn this argument into an ontology as this is already the extreme limit for his deconstructionist way of thinking.

2 "Patient thinker" is one of the terms Deleuze uses to refer to the "subject" in *Logic of Sense* and which quite fittingly highlights the often traumatizing impact of event on the subject that also in the same breath makes them a thinker. Deleuze began this usage in *Difference and Repetition* (Zourabichvili 56).

3 This argument is reminiscent of what Lacan postulates about the split of the subject into the subject of enunciation (the real) and the subject of statement (the symbolic or the world of language). In anticipation of possible criticisms on the psychoanalytical elements in this book, James Williams argues that "Deleuze goes beyond the particular content through his insistence of the role of the pure event and infinitives" (2008: 192) by quoting Deleuze: "It is only there [in metamorphosis, sublimation and symbolisation] that dying and killing, to castrate and to be castrated, to repair and to bring on, to wound and to withdraw, to devour and to be

devoured, to introject and to project, become pure events on the metaphysical surface that transforms them, where their infinitive is extracted" (Deleuze 2003: 221, 257). In fact, Deleuze himself is well informed of the mechanics of this split of the subject. In his "Cours Vincennes: dualism, monism and multiplicities", Deleuze elaborates on how this split has impelled us to submit to dualistic thinking and manipulations by authorities. And even though this was the period when Deleuze still took a strong interest in psychoanalysis, his theorization is already aimed at overcoming this dualism by means of among other things his undermining of language (Lecercle 2002: 250) and does not seem to need to rely on the concept of Oedipus as evidenced by the continuity from *Logic of Sense* to Deleuze's later works co-authored with Guattari. What is important here is the three stages distinguished in *Logic of Sense*: primary order, secondary organization, and tertiary arrangement, which do not necessarily pertain exclusively to the nuclear family. In any society where there is a rite of passage to adulthood, these stages exist.

4 The theme of "being forced to think" that develops explicitly from *Proust and Signs* (1964), through *Difference and Repetition* (1968) and *The Logic of Sense* (1969) to *Cinema 2* (1985), but also somewhat touched upon in his other books, basically revolves round the concept of sign, something enigmatic one encounters that disrupts one's current value system and prompts one to engage in genuine thinking. And the sign often takes the form of what Deleuze calls "style" or "non-style" that can "make language stutter" (Essays Critical and Clinical 113).

5 But the point is not to fall straight into the chaos but to institute a plane of immanence where the virtual possibilities can be available. Deleuze himself also takes pains to remind us that whereas the actualized crack instigates the counter-actualization, it is the latter that matters and therefore must take precedence lest the actualized crack would endanger the patient-thinker (LS 155–161).

6 The major figures in the OOO school have different and yet similar ways of naming the separation between the two dimensions of the object: Rift (Harman), gap (Bryant), and Rift/Wound (Morton). Timothy Morton explicitly tries to portray this rift as well as the "life" of an object in psychoanalytical terms (2013: 198–208).

7 "Prehension" is the term Whitehead uses to refer to the capacity in all objects, human or nonhuman, to "experience". Understood as "uncognitive apprehension" (Whitehead 1967: 69), prehension renders "the unity of a moment of experience" not contingent upon conscious operations (Vetlesen 2019: 75). In fact, agreeing with William James, Whitehead turns the much privileged "consciousness" into merely a "special element in the subjective forms of some feelings" (Whitehead 1978: 53). In other words, "consciousness presupposes experience, and not experience consciousness" (53). As a "mental activity", prehension "must be recognized as a property of everything that qualifies as real in Whitehead's sense" (Vetlesen 2019: 79–80) and "is one of the modes of feeling belonging to all actual events" (Whitehead 1978: 56). Thus, "all experience – throughout the entire continuum from the lowest to the highest level – begins with feelings or prehensions of other actual things, in which they grasp aspects of those things" (Vetlesen 2019: 86).

8 Jean-Jacques Lecercle makes a crucial distinction between what he calls the Deleuze event and the Badiou event. The former befouls one's cognition like a haze or mist whereas the latter upends the whole system of value like a volcanic eruption (2002: 109–118). But it seems to me that the Deleuze event can actually subsume both.

Bibliography

Ansell-Pearson, Keith. 1997. *The Viroid Life*. London: Routledge.

Bardini, Thierry. 2011. *Junkware*. Minneapolis: University of Minnesota Press.

Baudrillard, Jean. 2003. *The Spirit of Terrorism*. Brooklyn: Verso.
Beck, Christian and François-Xavier Gleyzon. 2016. 'Deleuze and the Event(s).' *Journal for Cultural Research*, 20(4): 329–333. https://doi.org/10.1080/14797585.2016.1264770
Bishop, Jeffrey P. and Martin J. Fitzgerald. 2020. 'Norming COVID-19: The Urgency of a Non-Humanist Holism.' *The Heythrop Journal*. https://doi.org/10.1111/heyj.13570
Borradori, Giovanna. 2003. *Philosophy in a Time of Terror: Dialogues with Jurgen Habermas and Jacques Derrida*. Chicago and London: The University of Chicago Press.
Boundas, Constantin. 2005. 'The Art of Begetting Monsters: The Unnatural Nuptials of Deleuze and Kant' in Stephen H. Daniel (ed.), *Current Continental Theory and Modern Philosophy*, 254–280. Evanston: Northwestern University Press.
Brunette, Peter and David Wills. 1989. *Screen/Play: Derrida and Film Theory*. Princeton and New Jersey: Princeton University Press.
Clark, Tim. 2008. "A Whiteheadian Chaosmos?" in Keith Robinson (ed.), *Deleuze, Whitehead, Bergson: Rhizomatic Connections*, 181–199. London: Palgrave Macmillan.
Deleuze, Gilles. 1973. *Cours Vincennes: Dualism, Monism and Multiplicities (Cours du 26/03/1973)*. Anti-Œdipe et Mille Plateaux. Translated by Daniel W. Smith. https://www.webdeleuze.com/textes/167
Deleuze, Gilles. 1988a. *Bergsonism*. Translated by Hugh Tomlinson. New York: Zone Books.
Deleuze, Gilles. 1988b. *Spinoza: Practical Philosophy*. Translated by Robert Hurley. San Francisco: City Light Books.
Deleuze, Gilles. 1989.*Cinema 2: The Time-Image*. Translated by Hugh Tomlinson and Robvert Galeta. Minneapolis: University of Minnesota Press.
Deleuze, Gilles. 1995a. *Difference and Repetition*. Translated by Paul Patton. New York: Columbia University Press.
Deleuze, Gilles. 1995b. *Negotiations 1972–1990*. Translated by Martin Joughin, New York: Columbia University Press.
Deleuze, Gilles. 1997a *Essays Critical and Clinical*. Translated by Daniel W. Smith and Michael A. Greco. London and New York: University of Minnesota Press.
Deleuze, Gilles. 1997b. "Immanence: A Life." *Theory, Culture & Society*, 14(2): 3–7. https://doi.org/10.1177/026327697014002002
Deleuze, Gilles. 2000. *Proust and Signs*. Translated by Richard Howard. London: The Athlone Press.
Deleuze, Gilles. 2003. *Francis Bacon: The Logic of Sensation*. Translated by Daniel W. Smith. London and New York: University of Minnesota Press.
Deleuze, Gilles and Felix Guattari. 1987. *A Thousand Plateaus: Capitalism and Schizophrenia*. Translated by Brian Massumi. London and New York: University of Minnesota Press.
Deleuze, Gilles and Felix Guattari. 2009. *Anti-Oedipus: Capitalism and Schizophrenia*. New York: Penguin.
Deleuze, Gilles and Felix Guattari. 1994. *What Is Philosophy?* Translated by Hugh Tomlinson and Graham Burchell. New York: Columbia University Press.
Grosz, Elizabeth. 2017. *The Incorporeal: Ontology, Ethics, and the Limits of Materialism*. New York: Columbia University Press.

Holland, Eugene. 2002. 'On Some Implications of Schizoanalysis.' *Strategies: Journal of Theory, Culture & Politics*, 15(1): 27–40. https://doi.org/10.1080/1040213022 0127834

Hughes, Joe. 2011. 'Believing in the World: Toward an Ethics of Form.' In Laura Guillaume and Joe Hughes (ed.), *Deleuze and the Body*, 73–95. Edinburgh: Edinburgh University Press.

Land, Christopher. 2005. "'Apomorphine Silence: Cutting-up Burroughs' Theory of Language and Control', *Ephemera: Theory and Politics in Organisation*, 5(3): 450–471. http://www.ephemerajournal.org/contribution/apomorphine-silence-cutting-burroughs-theory-language-and-control

Lapoujade, David. 2014. *Aberrant Movements: The Philosophy of Gilles Deleuze*. Translated by Joshua David Jordan. Paris: Semiotexe.

Lecercle, Jean-Jacques. 2002. *Deleuze and Language*. Basingstoke: Palgrave McMillan.

Markelj, Jernej. 2020. 'The Oedipal Bacillus: Contagion and Paranoia.' https://viral contagion.files.wordpress.com/2020/07/jernej_markelj_oedipal_bacillus.pdf

Marrati, Paola. 2008. *Gilles Deleuze: Cinema and Philosophy*. Translated by Alisa Hartz. Maryland: Johns Hopkins University Press.

Moelling, Karin and Felix Broecker. 2019. 'Viruses and Evolution – Viruses First? A Personal Perspective. *Frontiers in Microbiology* 10: 1–13, https://www.frontiersin.org/article/10.3389/fmicb.2019.00523

Morton, Timothy. 2013. *Realist Magic: Objects, Ontology, Causality*. Ann Arbor: Open Humanities Press.

Mythen, Gabe and Ulrich Beck. 2004. *A Critical Introduction to the Risk Society*. London: Pluto Press.

Neyrat, Frédéric. 2010. "The Birth of Immunopolitics." Translated by Arne De Boever. *Parrhesia: A Journal of Critical Philosophy*, 10: 31–38, www.parrhesia journal.org

Patton, Paul. 1997. 'The World Seen from Within: Deleuze and the Philosophy of Events.' *Theory & Event*, 1(1): 1–13. https://muse.jhu.edu/journals/theory_and_event/v001/1.1patton.html

Sellars, John. 2006. 'An Ethics of Event: Deleuze's Stoicisim.' *Angelaki: Journal of the Theoretical Humanities*, 11 (3): 151–171. https://doi.org/10.1080/096972506 01048622

Smith, Daniel and John Protevi. 2020. 'Gilles Deleuze' in Edward N. Zalta (ed.), *The Stanford Encyclopedia of Philosophy*, https://plato.stanford.edu/archives/spr2020/entries/deleuze/

Thiele, Kathrin. 2010. '"To Believe in This World, as It Is": Immanence and the Quest for Political Activism.' *Deleuze Studies* 4(Supp.): 28–45. https://doi.org/10.3366/dls.2010.0204

Vetlesen, Arne Johan. 2019. *Cosmologies of the Anthropocene: Panpsychism, Animism, and the Limits of Posthumanism*. London and New York: Routledge.

Villarreal, Luis P. and Guenther Witzany. 2010.'Viruses Are Essential Agents within the Roots and Stem of the Tree of Life.' *Journal of Theoretical Biology*, 262i(4): 698–710. https://doi.org/10.1016/j.jtbi.2009.10.014

Whitehead, Alfred North. 1978. *Process and Reality: An Essay in Cosmology*. New York: The Free Press.

Whitehead, Alfred North. 1967. *Science and the Modern World*. New York: The Free Press.

Williams, James. 2008. *Gilles Deleuze's Logic of Sense*. Edinburgh: Edinburgh University Press.
Williams, James. 2011. 'Never Too Late? On the Implications of Deleuze's Work on Death for a Deleuzian Moral Philosophy' in Nathan Jun and Daniel W. Smith (eds.), *Deleuze and Ethics*. Edinburgh: Edinburgh University Press, 171–187.
Zourabichvili, Francois. 1994. *Deleuze: The Philosophy of the Event*. Edinburgh: Edinburgh University Press.
Žukauskaitė, Audronė. 2014. 'The Schizoanalysis of Gilles Deleuze and Félix Guattari, or the Political between Schizophrenia and Paranoia' in Lene Auestad (ed.), *Nationalism and the Body Politic: Psychoanalysis and the Rise of Ethnocentrism and Xenophobia*, 109–126. New York: Routledge.

PART III

Thought in Response to the Pandemic

New Concepts

9

LIVING IN A WORLD WITHOUT OTHERS[1]

Gregg Lambert

The Three Robinsons

In the summer of 2020, amid the global pandemic, I decided to return to the fable of Robinson Crusoe to reflect on what it means to live in 'a world without others' (Deleuze). One morning I awoke on my own desert island and suddenly realized that despite all the critiques, from the early one by Horkheimer-Adorno to Derrida's more recent criticism of the 'Robinsonade' in philosophy, that *in (the) light of the pandemic* the very sense of the fable has changed and can no longer be dismissed as a mere fiction or colonial romance, but perhaps as the most literal approximation of real existence for many today. This is because, at least to some degree, everybody ('*tout le monde*' as the French have the habit of saying) has become a castaway and must learn to live in a world without others.

Nevertheless, I will not return to Defoe's original prototype of the fable, but instead to Michel Tournier's perverse avatar from the novel *Vendredi, ou les limbes du Pacifique* (1967). Of course, there is a much simpler explanation as to why I choose Tournier's version over Defoe's, since it is the only version of the story of Robinson Crusoe that I brought with me to my own desert island. Therefore, one must make do with whatever one has at hand. This oversight has also proved to be opportune since, in my view, Defoe's Robinson Crusoe never actually experienced his own shipwreck, and never really departed from the world of others, since he brought his culture and religion with him – packed in watertight compartments in the large suitcases he rescued from the *Virginia* – and so in this regard he was more of a colonizer than a castaway.

DOI: 10.4324/9781003507789-12

To picture the extreme situation of living in a world without others, therefore, demands more than a simple desert island fable, but a more phenomenological investigation of the subject of Robinson himself. As Tournier's version exemplifies, first, to be 'alone,' there must also be others, or what Deleuze refers to in his commentary on the novel as an *a priori* Other, or an 'Other-Structure,' that in many ways resembles Heidegger's description of the world that is populated by others as a complete structure of references and referrals (*verweisungen*) that constitute the very possibility of subjectivity. I can only be alone apart from all the others, or at a remote distance from the world of others; otherwise, solitude would never be experienced as *my own*. However, given the extreme state of solitude that is being suffered by many castaways locked into their private apartments or separate rooms, with or without the company of a companion animal or a Friday, I decided to choose Tournier's version of the fable to explore whether, ontologically speaking, it is possible to speak of a world without others, or of an existence without world, and remain 'I' or 'oneself'.

Taking up my claim that the *fabula* of Robinson Crusoe has changed sense today, if only because, at least to some degree, everybody (*tout le monde*) is living on a desert island, this is not intended as an empirical description of the many different states of affairs caused by the pandemic or by the underlying inequalities of global populations. Instead, it is only a statement that one no longer needs a fable to imagine the existential reality of such an 'extreme situation' of solitude. Sometimes it is necessary to place an ocean between yourself and the world of others to reflect on your existence, but the idea that one can choose to become a castaway one day is nothing but a fiction. Nevertheless, the fiction of the desert island still serves a useful and dialectical function as a surface of reflection on existence, which cannot be viewed directly – at least, not at first. (It is a bit like what Plato said about the sun, which can only be viewed in the reflection that appears in a puddle of water.) After all, why do we read novels to look at our own existence? To gain the necessary vantage-point? To look at ourselves from a second or third perspective point of view? In this sense, the fable functions as a navigational beacon homing in on the world that was once populated by others, which is now called 'the former world', or the world that is gone.

Once again, this recalls Heidegger's earlier definition of signs – and what are novels but a certain constellation of signs? – as 'equipment' for referring to or showing something else (*Verweisung*), and he also pointed to the way the sign's own phenomenological aspect immediately disappears in referring to something in its place. Is this not also to define the function of a novel as a kind of equipment for causing our familiar existence to become visible and, at the same time, strangely unfamiliar (*unheimlich*), that is, to give it the status of a shadow or a refection? This is the ontological status of all fiction. And yet, according to the term of my claim that the ontological sense of the

Robinson fable has changed *in (the) light of the pandemic*, what use will we have for the fable now? This will be the subject of my investigation.

Concerning the fact that the prototypical Crusoe was never really exposed to the extreme situation we are imagining today, this has been noted before by many others. It was first observed by Ian Watt in *The Rise of the Novel*, who perceived in the description of Robinson Crusoe's neat and tidy island, in which everything has a place and there is a place for everything, the perfect representation of the mode of production and the relations between production and consumption that prefigure the emergence modern capitalism, including a certain Protestant temperament of the dry and completely humourless type of liberal individual that Crusoe represented, a real 'bore'. As Deleuze once commented, if there is an upside to the fact that children are still forced to read the most boring novel in the world, perhaps it can be found in the completely healthy reaction that it might provoke in them to avoid becoming such an individual themselves.

However, it was Virginia Woolf who first perceived in Defoe's own alter-ego the sad domestic economy of a typical English gentleman, whose ideal intimate companion would be a dog curled up at his feet, and a boy, rather than a member of the opposite sex, who would later turn out to be Robinson's 'Man Friday' in the *Farther Adventures* (Woolf 1994: 283-287). In other words, Woolf immediately discerned that Defoe didn't need to travel at all to find Robinson Crusoe's island, and that the South Sea adventure was merely a popular fictional vehicle that Defoe had ripped off from the London newspapers of this period to portray the external space of his own desert island subjectivity. As Defoe himself confessed in *Serious Observations*, one does not actually need a desert island, since 'I never feel myself more alone than in the center of a populous city like London'.[2] It is a lasting historical irony that Crusoe's desert island was England itself, an island populated by smaller islands.

The South African novelist JM Coetzee would later deploy Woolf's insight in his own version, *Foe*, which is the story of a female castaway, Susan Barton, who narrowly escaped the abuse of Brazilian slavers by slipping overboard in the middle of the night and ending up on the island with the actual 'Cruso' and, of course, Friday, 'a Negro with a head of fuzzy wool, naked except for a pair of drawers' (Coetzee 1986: 1). Nevertheless, Coetzee employs the fable as an allegory of a colonial Afrikaans woman writer who travels to London to confront the famous author, Daniel Foe, for plagiarizing her own castaway narrative, and ends up occupying the author's apartments in Kensington while Foe is in prison for unpaid debts, bringing along her shadow, the black and mute figure of Friday. When the author finally returns, Barton holds him hostage and forces him to acknowledge the dubious existence of certain letters she wrote to the author recounting her misfortune and her encounter with the real 'Cruso,' that is, to admit to the fact that this was really *her story*, and it was moreover real and not simply a fable invented by her 'Foe' (enemy). As an aside, even though Derrida (2020) mentions the novel in his own reading of the Robinson fable in *The Beast and the Sovereign*, he apparently never read more than the title, especially in the claim that there is 'no trace of woman' (*Pas trace de femme*) on Crusoe's Island – and thus could be accused along with the author himself for eliding the existence of *a real female castaway*. Ultimately, Coetzee's version gradually strips away all allegorical representation and destroys the fable itself by revealing the finger of a 'darker author' who is writing on the wall of colonial history, the real Friday who will seal the fate of the castaways, Daniel Foe and Susan Barton (Coetzee 1986: 134).

Turning now to Tournier's version of the fable, the reader might already have guessed that it narrates the experience of another (*autrui*) Robinson, and most importantly for our purposes, describes the possible transformative and even destructive effects of living in a world without others, which is why I have decided to employ its fable either as a word of warning or sign of hope for the reader and fellow castaway. The novel begins, prior to the shipwreck, with the fortune telling of 'Robinson's' fate as told through a reading of tarot cards by Captain Van Deyssel. As the captain says, 'my brief lecture is in some sort of a coded message, and the key to the cipher is your future itself' (Tournier 1997: 13). Each card represents a different stage of Robinson's solitude, from the loss of his original identity due to the corrosive effects of his estrangement from the world of others to the eventual recovery of a new subjectivity caused by his union with the quasi-mythical being of Friday.

The first card reveals the Demiurge, the creator of second order; 'there is an organizer in you,' says the captain, 'one who does battle with a world in disorder which he seeks to master by whatever means come to his hand' (Tournier 1997: 8). 'Mars,' said the captain. 'The little Demiurge has achieved a seeming victory over Nature. He has triumphed by the force of his own will and imposed an order which is in his own image' (Tournier 1997: 8). With these words, the captain stops to reflect upon Robinson's own image to imagine what this world might look like:

> Robinson the King ... you are 22. You have deserted – that is to say, left behind in York – a young wife and two children, to seek your fortune in the new world, like so many of your compatriots. Your close-cropped hair and square, russet beard, clear eyed steady gaze, in which there is a hint of something narrow and rigid, your attire, whose sobriety is near to affectation – all this puts you in the category of those who never had doubts. You are pious, parsimonious, pure.
>
> *(Tournier 1997: 9)*

Through the voice of the Captain, Tournier parodies the portrait of Defoe's original prototype as a young colonizer. If there is a dominant psychological trait that appears in the Captain's words, it is the perception of Robinson's anal character, which will play an important part in the re-creation of the new house economy on his island. 'The kingdom over which you will preside will be like one of those tidy cupboards where the women of our country keep their piles of immaculate linen scented with lavender' (Tournier 1997: 9). At this point, as the reader might have expected, the captain prophesizes Robinson's 'downgoing' (*Untergangen*), which comes from Nietzsche's *Thus Spoke Zarathustra* but also echoes the Heideggerian theme of 'thrownness' and coming face to face with the 'nothing' of the world (Heidegger 1962: 321). However, the true cause of Robinson's descent was already implicit in the judgment that underlies the captain's sarcasm: Robinson is inexperienced, a heterosexual white male of twenty-two, even though Robinson himself is – at the moment of his tarot reading –completely unconscious of his inexperience and carelessness towards others, such as his wife and children who he left behind to go on his adventure. (In the original novel, Crusoe's father even forewarns the young adventurer of the catastrophe that will befall him as God's judgment for his desire to escape his 'station in life' and, in the end, would become 'the most Miserable wretch that ever was born') (Defoe 1994: 5–6). Only the immanent shipwreck will reveal to Robinson the fact of the captain's final judgment: 'The truth is you have everything to learn' (Tournier 1997: 8).

On the island, immediately following the shipwreck, Robinson begins to learn the reality of his extreme solitude. The first effect of solitude that Robinson notices is an immediate distortion of the perceptual field: 'Optical illusions, mirages, hallucinations, waking dreams, imagined sounds, fantasy and delirium ....' (Tournier 1997: 54). This also has immediate effects upon Robinson's natural capacity for speech, or 'actualised language.' 'Language,' according to Robinson's logbook, 'in a fundamental manner evokes a peopled world, where the others like so many lamps casting a glow of light around them in which everything is, if not known, at least knowable. The lights have vanished from my consciousness' (Tournier 1997: 55). In fact, by the time that Friday arrives on the island in Tournier's version, the power of language – the identity of the subject that it brings with it, along with the community to which this subject belongs – has atrophied to the point where words themselves appear more like dream images. All associations appear false or strangely distorted, and consciousness longer glows with the illumination of interiors and the contours usually furnished by others.

Only after a brief period on the island, Robinson's own body is no longer defined as a 'possession' of Robinson himself but appears to resemble a 'Thing' in a neutral and objective relation to other bodies or objects which are either present or found to be missing from the reality of the island. Robinson's own perception of his own body is reduced to being purely 'present to hand' (*Vorhandeln*) like a common object merely expressing the predicate relationship of 'the body of Robinson,' but with no more proximity to the subject than statements like 'Robinson's pipe,' or 'Robinson's goat'. In other words, the predicate relationship that language usually expresses is now contingent and can undergo further modification as, for example, when a common object (e.g., my comb, my keys) is accidentally lost or destroyed. By the end of this process, Robinson gradually sheds all the attributes of his former identity such as age, gender, race, sexuality, nationality, memory, perception: in short, the subject of 'Robinson' is peeled like an onion and vanishes, layer by layer.

As the duration of Robinson's solitude on the island grows longer, Tournier describes a state in which Robinson's consciousness begins to merge with the island itself, a process that is accompanied by Robinson's descent into the inner core of 'Speranza' and the discovery of a secret coombe where he curls up and goes to sleep. In a later journal entry, Robinson himself comments on the significance of the last barrier of his subjectivity that has been dismantled by his experience of solitude. It is at this moment that Robinson compares his state to the conscious recognition of his own physical death in the consciousness of others.

> All those who knew me, all without exception, believe me dead. My own belief in my existence is opposed to that of unanimous belief. No matter what I do, I cannot prevent that picture of Robinson's dead body from existing in all their minds. This alone, although certainly it does not kill me, suffices to remove me to the outermost confines of life, to a place hung between heaven and hell--in a word, to a Limbo.
>
> *(Tournier 1997: 123)*

We might understand this comparison as a more accelerated duration of natural death that is usually made visible by a fatal disease but otherwise operates invisibly and imperceptibly in the individual's body from the moment of birth. In the foregoing quotation, the mechanism that causes this accelerated state of decomposition is the association of Robinson's name with the picture of Robinson's dead body, which initiates a gradual fading of the distinct presence of Robinson to himself 'in the minds of these Others'. Of course, what this implies is that the only thing that was holding Robinson's former identity together while he was alive was the very same structure of association that actually originated from the presence of others; therefore, the gradual release of the others' grip on Robinson's presence-to-himself positively frees him from being *Robinson-himself*, who was, in fact, only *Robinson-for-the-others*.

Nevertheless, this positive discovery also constitutes the revelation of the identity of death and sexuality in Robinson's consciousness. On the sea floor surrounding the island (Robinson's body), a small crevice occurs and suddenly widens, where the earth is ripped open. At first a canyon appears from the small crack of Robinson's anus and tidal waves spill over the entire surface of the island. The first wave would be a shift that occurs in the meaning of Robinson's solitude, which he initially enjoys with his bride 'Speranza' (the earth) by crawling into the dark recesses of her body to deposit his seed in the 'pink coombe'. Nevertheless, the danger lurking in Robinson's sexual union with Speranza is his continued vulnerability to all manners of 'wallowing in the mire,' which Freud had attributed to the persistence of the 'death instinct' (*Todestrieb*). In other words, surviving the disequilibrium caused by the fear of his natural death, Robinson has managed only to construct a state of affairs that is even further from equilibrium. Thus, he will only be saved from this second death, an inorganic death much more terrifying than the natural death he has just survived by the intervention of Friday.

Who is Robinson's Friday? In Tournier's version, Friday represents nothing more than the reality principle that threatens to deconstruct the fragile order that Robinson constructs by means of his sexual union with Speranza. Thus, from the very beginning, Friday's very presence on the island seems to disturb the order and tidiness of Robinson's, and his actions fundamentally disturb its strictly economic and prescribed order of days and places, as well as the moral codes of propriety and impropriety that were far too rigidly ordered, like the 'tidy cupboard of immaculate linen scented with lavender' that was earlier prophesied by the Captain. At the same time, the introduction of Friday's presence already foreshadows a new understanding of desire that is no longer founded by the notions of possession and property that belonged to Robinson's previous economic arrangements of heterosexual desire. As I have already outlined, the first economic determination of the sexual object was destroyed by the corrosive effects of Robinson's solitude caused by his estrangement from the others. The second economic arrangement reproduces itself by transferring Robinson's desire for a lost or missing sexual object onto the body of Speranza herself. Reflecting on a dream in his journal, Robinson eventually concludes that both these earlier failures were caused by the residual elements of anthropomorphism that still influenced the sexual organization of his substance.

> My love affair with Speranza was still largely human in its nature. I fecundated her soil as though I were lying with a wife. It was Friday who brought about a deeper change. The harsh stab of desire that pierces the loins of the lover has been transformed for me into a soft jubilation which exalts and pervades me from head to foot, so long as the sun-god bathes me from head to foot.
>
> *(Tournier 1997: 212)*

Finally, the foregoing dream-work prefigures a last phase where Robinson's sexuality undergoes another and final metamorphosis, as was foretold in the tarot reading where the combination of Robinson-Friday prefigures the arrival of a new avatar of Venus 'rising from the waves'. It represents the culmination of the series of metamorphoses that Robinson's 'substance' undergoes that lead to a final teleological accord with a pure and elemental Desire, which is described as the coupling of Friday and Robinson who are born from '*le Grand Luminaire Halluciné*,' the moon goddess who has swept the stars from the night sky (*désastré*). At this point, Robinson is writing in his journal or dream-diary by the light of the moon while Friday is curled up like a blossom or an egg at Robinson's feet. In this state of enraptured vision, Robinson is finally able to sink all the way to 'the hither side of consciousness' and slip his yoke into the egg of Friday's hallucinatory presence:

> Vague patterns appear and vanish on the white disc, shadowy hands reach and clasp, faces smile for an instant, to vanish into mist. The spinning gains in speed until it resembles immobility, as though the very excess of turbulence had caused the lunar jelly to set. And gradually the pattern is defined. There are two poles at either end of the egg, with a tracing of lines between them. The poles become heads, and the arabesque the outline of two conjoined bodies. Two similar beings, twins, are in the process of gestation: Gemini are being born on the moon
>
> *(Tournier 1997: 213)*

In the foregoing passage, Tournier reveals the identity of Friday as the avatar of Robinson's sexual metamorphosis. Friday appears in the waves in the figure of Venus who 'drives Robinson out into the region of her father Uranus' and returns them to a state of pure and elemental sexuality, one that neither colonizes the earth nor requires a detour through the body of woman: '*The truth is that the height to which we have soared, Friday and I, the difference between the sexes has been surpassed …*' (Tournier 1997: 230). Robinson is now 'a Uranian,' so that when a ship finally appears and then departs, it does not return home with Robinson (who by now has lost all filiation with his former species), but rather Friday who travels back to Europe in Robinson's place. In Friday's place there suddenly appears a new cast-away, an orphaned child who steals away from the presence of the sailors in the middle of the night to live with Robinson (a bit like Susan Barton in Coetzee's version). This is the child who Robinson will adopt as his new companion. Since he comes from Estonia and his name, 'Jaan Neljapäev,' is unpronounceable, Robinson decides to name him 'Tuesday,' since '*Tuesday is the Sunday of children*' (Tournier 1997: 254).

Concluding my brief précis of the fable, if I said earlier on that Tournier's version is a more realistic account of the extreme situation of living on a desert island than Defoe's original narrative, I would now qualify this statement by saying that this only extends to the account of Robinson's initial effects of solitude (which is more or less accurate, speaking from personal experience). However, beginning with the arrival of the child Friday, and all the metamorphoses that Robinson undergoes from that moment onward, the novel is more like science fiction in the fantastical account of the hallucinatory phenomena caused by Robinson's loss of the world of others. As to the real cause of the hallucinations, I can only speculate, but perhaps he ate some wild berries on the island that produced the same psychotropic effects as LSD, including the final vision of Friday as Venus rising from the waves. Nevertheless, what this illustrates is that both the extreme poles of depressive and schizoid mania must also be recognized as possible 'existential attunements' (Heidegger), alongside the normal effects of profound boredom and insomnia, for the purposes of our phenomenological investigation of solitude. A second hypothesis would be that everything that transpires following what I will define as Robinson's schizoid and depressive phases takes place deep in the cave where Robinson is dreaming, and thus everything afterward – including the arrival of Friday, and later, the child Tuesday – is part of the long dream that begins when the conscious Robinson falls unconscious.

Regardless, there are only two possible endings to any castaway narrative: rescue or death. Concerning the ending of Tournier's narrative, therefore, either we must imagine Robinson curled up in the deepest part of his cave dreaming of the events incidents involving metamorphosis with Friday, as well as the ship that eventually lands on the island to take Friday away and deposit Jaan Neljapäev, who becomes the new child Tuesday; or, we must imagine Robinson Crusoe already dead and what we have been reading is the dream-dairy that was salvaged from the cave. If this were indeed the case, then Coetzee's ending of the novel *Foe* is perhaps more realistic in showing the bloated corpses of Susan Barton, the female castaway, and Daniel Foe, the author, floating in the stateroom of the *Virginia*. Circling above them, on the ceiling of their sunken crypt, is the dark shadow of Friday on a bamboo raft, throwing flowers on their watery grave. (In applying this fable to the present, perhaps our own ending will be no different.)

The Schizoid and Depressive Poles

In an early essay that first appeared in 1967 and was published as an appendix to *Logique du sens* (1969), '*Michel Tournier et le monde sans Autrui*,' Gilles Deleuze (1969: 352) employs Tournier's 'philosophical novel' to pose the following question: 'must we conclude that sexuality is the only fantastic principle able to bring about a deviation from the rigorous economic order assigned by the origin?'[3]

This question must be understood in two senses, the first of which requires a radical revision of Heidegger's concept of world as a 'whole structure' and the role of others as constituent parts of this structure by incorporating the fundamental component of sexuality in what Deleuze calls the 'Other-Structure.' Why? Because, in the case of Heidegger's ontology, one can easily apply Derrida's earlier claim that there is 'no trace of woman' (*Pas trace de Femme*) – actually, no trace of any sexuality whatsoever! The second sense of the question, which I will return to at the end, concerns replacing sexual difference at the origin of human subjectivity with what he and Guattari later call 'becoming' (as in 'becoming-woman,' 'becoming-animal,' becoming molecular,' etc.) – that is to say, to replace sexual difference as an origin with the deviation from normative sexuality as a 'final end,' that is, in analogy to a psychoanalytic understanding of the goal of perversion. Corresponding to both senses of the foregoing question, Deleuze employs Tournier's version of Robinson as an 'instrument of research' to investigate the effects of the absence of the Other-Structure in the extremely artificial situation of the fable of another Robinson. As Deleuze (1969: 354) writes, 'philosophical reflection can benefit from what the novel shows with so much force and life'.

First, what Tournier's novel reveals is the crucial role that the presence of the Other-Structure plays in the entire 'organization' of the world from its margin or background, the transitions from one field of perception to the next. In short, the presence of Others already attests to a structural organization of the world in both itself and in its margins, but it also operates the possible transitions from the unseen depths of the subject's own body to the visible surfaces of objects. Drawing in part on Sartre's phenomenological analysis of the Other in *Being and Nothingness*, Deleuze describes the normal functioning of the perceptual field that is conditioned by the presence of others as follows:

> The part of the object I do not see I posit as visible to others; so when I will have walked around to reach this hidden part, I will have joined up with the others behind the object to create a totalization I had already anticipated. And as for the objects behind my back, I sense them coming together to form a world, precisely because they are visible to, and are seen by, others. [...] In short, the others assure the margins and transitions in the world.
>
> *(Deleuze 1969: 355)*

Contrary to Sartre's earlier analysis, however, Deleuze argues that this crucial phenomenological significance only comes into view from the effects artificially produced in the novel by the absence of actual others. (In some ways this claim also corresponds to Heidegger's central argument in *Being and Time* concerning the disruption that may occur in the whole structure of the world through the damage or loss of one of its constituent parts.) For example, if we recall the effects caused by the immediate absence of others from

Robinson's consciousness in the initial phase of his solitude on the island, they are described as: *'Optical illusions, mirages, hallucinations, waking dreams, imagined sounds, fantasy and delirium …'* (Tournier 1997: 54). These effects occur as a direct result of the absence of an Other-Structure that is normally actualized through the concrete presence of others, causing the relationship between depth, margin, and center in perception-consciousness to fundamentally become disoriented and disorganized.

Second, I have already recounted the gradual transformation of the phenomenological sense attached to Robinson's own body, which becomes merely a neutral object among other objects on the island. In addition, there is also a sense of the violent dispossession of the body's own sexual organization that is the direct result of the absence of others and touches on the struggle between the depths of Robinson's body and the surface that was formerly organized by genital sexuality, specifically the crucial role played by the 'good object' that is suddenly discovered to be missing or lost altogether. Here, we should recall the captain's earlier description of the 22-year-old Robinson who has left a wife and children at home in England. Most contemporary theories of the 'Other' assume that the attributes of sexuality or race are fundamental components of the Other-Structure; however, this is far from certain and predicated on the assumption that the essential attributes of subjectivity are 'thing-like,' present-to-hand, and readily visible to others (an assumption that is not only pre-phenomenological but strangely pre-Cartesian, which is to say, onto-theological). On this point, I choose to remain strictly Heideggerian.

Third, I have already spoken about the gradual fading of Robinson's relationship to his own body as a subjective property (i.e., the phenomenological sense of 'having a body that is mine'), but this is also clearly revealed in Robinson's experience of his own nakedness, which undergoes an even more fundamental estrangement. During his self-described periods of 'wallowing in the mire,' Robinson is defined as the 'excrement of Speranza' and often sleeps and defecates without any concern for cleanliness or propriety, which can only exist as a subjective form of concern (or 'care' in the Heideggerian sense of *Sorge*). Thus, the state of 'being naked' is more extreme than the nudity that only addresses the relative relationship of the body's depths and surfaces always from the perspective of the world of others. Rather, Tournier describes the experience of nakedness as a severe exposure to the depths of the body, or as a return to an inorganic substance, as the extreme point of de-subjectivation.

> Nakedness is a luxury in which a man may indulge himself without danger only when he is warmly surrounded by his fellow man. For Robinson, while his soul has not yet undergone any change, it was a trial of desperate temerity. Stripped of its threadbare garments – worn, tattered, and sullied,

> but the fruit of civilized millennia, and impregnated with human associations – his vulnerable body was at the mercy of every hostile element.
>
> *(Tournier 1997: 33)*

Eventually, Robinson's former body is reduced to being an empty surface of pure sensation to every painful blow, every collision, every encounter with objects and other bodies in a flat and desubjectivized space of pure relations. In many ways, this also recalls Emmanuel Levinas' description of a purely impersonal and anonymous plane of Being, of the 'there is' *(il y a)* described as the 'horror' of a nocturnal space where there is neither object nor even the profile of an object, but rather only as 'a swarming of points' that do not refer to one another as in illuminated space, since there is no perspective either (Levinas 2013: 83). The question we need to ask is what this existential attunement of 'horror' that comes from the depths of the body have to do with the surface constituted by sexuality, and what is the relationship of this surface to what Deleuze calls the 'Other-Structure'?

Employing the psychoanalytic theories of Freud and Melanie Klein (as well as Lacan's theory of the 'Symbolic,' which is an essential component in Deleuze's own conception of the 'Other-Structure'), Deleuze reorients the role played by sexuality in the organization of the relation between the depths of the body produced by the primary processes and the partial surfaces or 'territories' produced by the organization of genital sexuality. The construction of the erogenous zones on the body results from the creation of a pure surface that does not have, on its underside, the depth of the body filled with partial objects; rather, the other side of the surface is comprised by the absence of the lost or missing object that is completely separate from the depths and situated in the field of the Other, according to the well-known Lacanian formulation that 'Human desire *is* Other-desire'. Recalling Lacan's famous description of the 'Mirror stage' that precedes the organization of sexuality – and the genital organization, in particular – it is the ego's jubilant assumption of its own ideal image that becomes the prototype for this separation and subsequent 'alienation' (*aphanasis*) of a lost or missing object, namely, the ego's own *imago* which can be defined as a pure surface upon which the sexual determination of the 'good object' will come to be reflected at a later stage.

Following Klein's insistence on the positive and 'reparative' role of the formation of the surfaces produced by the organization of genital sexuality, Deleuze also highlight the function of the phallus defined as the image of the good object projected on the genital zone of the 'Body without Organs' as 'restorative' of a surface that mends and protects the ego itself from the destructive drives that are constantly and violently pushed back into the depths of the body. (In short, the body without organs is literally stitched up so that the body's orifices are closed by the erogenous zones to prevent the depths of the body from leaking out.) 'Above all,' Deleuze writes, 'it is here that the child pursues on his own body the constitution of a surface and the integration of the erogenous zones, thanks to the well-founded privilege of the genital zone' –something, I would add, that occurs repeatedly throughout the subject's sexual life, especially when the object is repeatedly discovered to be missing, stolen away, or lost altogether (Deleuze 1969: 221). Therefore, it is only from the 'depressive position' that results from the loss of the good object and the surface that was formerly constituted by genital sexuality that Deleuze will deduce the crucial role that sexuality plays in constructing his own theory of the 'Other-Structure'.

At this point, recalling Tourner's account of Robinson's own depression after the discovery of the lost or missing object of sexual desire, the first effect of the absence of the Other-Structure is the return of the depths constituted by the oral and the anal drives and the alimentary and excremental partial objects that are introjected into the ego's own body, but also and more crucially into the bodies of others where they will function as the ego's own partial objects. Deleuze will interpret this first moment as a regression to what Klein called the paranoid-schizoid position and the return of the fragmented body composed of partial objects of the drives. It is here we discover the real 'horror' of the drives, including the paranoid feelings of being persecuted by the bad introjected objects of the depths and hallucinatory visions that rise to the surface of consciousness in dreams. These are the manifestations of the partial objects that are *either* introjected and restrained in the depths of the body by the organization of genital sexuality, *or* they projected into the bodies of others where they are aggressively pursued and persecuted – *especially in the body of the mother, which becomes the prototype for the paranoid-schizoid aggressiveness that the ego will project onto all future sexual relations.*

For example, we might recall that in Defoe's original version, Crusoe is initially overcome by anxiety and paranoid fear of being eaten by predators or cannibals which represents the return the paranoid-schizoid aggressiveness of the infantile oral drive. In Tournier's version, however, recalling the captain's astute diagnosis of Robinson's anal-erotic character, we the effects of the return of the anal drive results in Robinson's body being turned into excrement. *'He relieved himself where he lay, and rarely failed to roll in the damp warmth of his own excrement. He moved less and less, and his brief ended in his return to the depths of the mire ... only his eyes, nose, and mouth were active, alert for edible weed and toad spawning drifting on the surface'* (Tournier 1997: 40). As an aside, the role played by the drives and their partial objects might provide an alternative ontological account of the origin of what Heidegger called 'moods,' and particularly anxiousness (*Sichängsten*). Of course, Heidegger himself would never accept the 'ontic' theory of the primordial role of the drives in infantile consciousness as even a partial explanation of what he calls the 'pre-ontological' character of existential moods.

Returning to the second phase of Robinson's depressive position, this is represented by all his attempts to recover the missing or lost object by projecting it onto the surface of the island that has now replaced Robinson's own ego. Accordingly, this phase represents the depressive position proper that succeeds the manic-schizoid position of the drives and their partial and introjected objects and, which again, represented Robinson's attempt to 'repair' the surface that was lost in the previous schizoid stage and was caused by the initial 'disorganization' of genital sexuality. For example, in the pages of the books that had been erased by the tides and bleached by the sun, Robinson begins to create a new organization for the surface of Speranza, constructing articles of government, polity, penal systems, calendars, days of fasting and celebration, ritual forms of internment, burial, and commemoration. The fact that all this work of restoration of the surface appears to take place from a 'a great height,' as if from a bird's eye view of the island itself, is significant in showing the new distance from the depths of the body that are affected by the superficial order that Robinson now constructs on the surface of the island itself. As Deleuze writes: 'Height, in fact, has a strange power of reaction to the depths. It seems, from the point of height, that depth turns, orients itself in a new manner, and spreads itself; from a bird's eye view, it is but a fold easily undone, or rather a local orifice surrounded or stitched to the surface' (Deleuze 1969: 223). Nevertheless, the organization of surfaces constructed from the depressive position usually succumb to failure in the end, causing the ego to crash back into the infinite depths of the body, that is, its continued vulnerability to all manners of 'wallowing in the mire.'

At this point in his interpretation of the fable, however, Deleuze departs from both Freud and Klein by arguing that a more profound 'splitting' (*Spaltung)* of the subject transcends the division between the depths of the body constituted by the drives and their partial objects and the partial surfaces of the erogenous zones constituted by the sexual objects (including any number of the arrangements of genital sexuality that are produced by the perversions). In fact, the real struggle detected in the reaction of the depressive position is between the depths of a body containing the explosive, noxious, and threatening introjected and projected internal objects and what Deleuze calls a 'body without organs and without mechanisms renouncing both projection and introjection' that is produced primarily as a means of protecting the ego from its own body composed of both organs *and* partial objects. This will lead him to the discovery of a third position, which Deleuze calls 'the sexual-perverse,' and can be defined by the autonomy proper to the organization of its own surfaces and erogenous zones in the relative absence or negation of the 'Other-Structure'. In other words, it is the relative autonomy of the organization of surfaces composed of erogenous zones that already prefigures the possible separation of the ego itself as the 'body without organs,' which is now opposed to the bodies produced by the depths of the schizoid position and the partial surfaces constructed by the depressive position: a body that takes the ego itself for the 'good object' and, more importantly for our purposes, substitutes for the original organization of genital sexuality an *anorganic form of immanent desire that no longer requires the detour through another body.*

It is around the 'goal' represented by this third position that we can now return Deleuze's question of 'becoming' that psychoanalysis has only understood negatively as the symptomatic role of the perversions in resisting the normative function of the Other-Structure. Following the orientation of Klein, Deleuze assigns perversion a more positive and potentially transformative role: rather than repairing or reconstructing the broken or damaged surfaces of the body constructed by the erogenous zones, the sexual-perverse position attempts to bypass the origin of sexuality difference altogether and to replace this origin with another goal – that of becoming '*otherwise than the other sex!*' If we examine the 'becoming' of Friday-Robinson represented by the third metamorphosis, the first things we should notice is that Robinson has managed to bypass the paranoid-schizoid position of the drives that had dominated in the first stage, but also the manic-depressive position in the second stage, since this was too dependent on the subjugation of an external body (first, the body of woman, and then the body of Speranza herself, the earth). As Robinson claims: *'The truth is that the height to which we have soared, Friday and I, the difference between the sexes has been surpassed …'* (Tournier 1997: 230). At this point in the fable, the formerly separated bodies of Robinson and Friday spinning in a white disc until the yoke of Robinson's former body is blended with Friday's yoke, and the single body of Robinson-Friday exhibits 'the beauty of glass and metal and of shining surfaces, a glitter that does not belong to living things' (Tournier 1997: 213). Finally, once the goal of Robinson-Friday's becoming is achieved, all the sadness and loss that originally belonged to sexuality is now completely surpassed by what Deleuze now calls (for the first time, I believe) a complete 'Body without Organs.' *'Voila!'* Deleuze writes, 'this is Robinson's final discovery: discovery of the pure surface, of an elemental beyond, of an 'otherwise than another' (*L'Autre qu'autrui*)' (Deleuze 1969: 370).

This represents the radical Nietzscheanism of Deleuze's moral question concerning the 'fantastic principle' of perversion, which was intended to release the surface produced by fantasy from its secondary and derivative position in the organization of 'desiring economy' (i.e., Oedipus). It is this positive discovery of a complete body with organs composed of pure elements and surfaces that explains why Deleuze, even in his earlier commentary on the subject of masochism, often claims a positive and transformative role for phantasy as the 'virtual' production of desire that expresses a substance of becoming rather than original organic determination of substance by the instincts as in Freud. Nevertheless, this expression of 'becoming' is normally demoted to servicing the imaginary, where the productive and potentially transformative nature of desire is always trapped by the different genital organizations of sexuality that must always refer to the 'Other-Structure' for their actualization. In other words, the plane constituted by desire must also detour through the framework of institutions and myths for the most common fantasies that populate the 'Other-Structure' – as in the case of the myth of Oedipus and certainly in the case of the fable of Robinson Crusoe! Consequently, the sexual-perverse position risks producing yet another post-Oedipal myth of the same conflict between the depressive and schizoid poles that serves to organize the drives and their partial objects, which is why Deleuze also observes that the body without organs it produces often appears as a 'sterile double' of the 'Other-Structure'.

Finally, at the conclusion of his own research on the question of whether perversion can offer us the 'fantastic principle' that will convert sexual difference as an origin into the goal of becoming 'Otherwise than the other sex,' Deleuze must now also acknowledge that the price one must pay for the liberation of a pure and elemental desire is the murder of both the 'Other' and of all 'the others'. Thus, the ultimate goal of 'all perversion is an 'Other-cide' and an 'altruicide' (Deleuze 1969: 370). Moreover, when the 'Other-Structure' is found to be completely absent or somehow negated by purely artificial means, henceforth the only role that 'real "others" can play, in the second structure, is the role of bodies-victims, bodies-doubles, or the role of accomplice-doubles, or the role of accomplices-elements' (Deleuze 1969: 371). For example, recalling the third metamorphosis of the fable, it would no longer be even accurate to say that Robinson and Friday can become others to each other since the whole 'Other Structure' is now gone, and along with it the possibility of another and of all the others! What has taken their place are pure *simulacra*, that is, pure doubles or twins created to serve a new plane of immanence that assumed the ultimate goal of Robinson's image of 'Great Health,' the plane of immanent desire that is produced by a return to primary narcissism.

However, even more troubling are what I have already alluded to earlier as other existential attunements that can be associated with a situation of extreme solitude, attunements of desire that demand nothing less than the sacrifice of the organic body itself as the price one must ultimately pay for producing a complete body without organs. This is true for the body without organs that is produced by alcoholism, certain drug addictions, and naturally, suicide – *and it is certainly true in most of cases involving the body without organs produced by real psychosis and real schizophrenia*! Finally, because he must acknowledge that these dangers also define a process of 'becoming' that replaces *an origin* with *a goal*, Deleuze must also conclude that certain 'becomings' cannot exist in a world of others, since the world created in the absence of others is composed of an atmosphere that expresses 'a strange Spinozism lacking any oxygen in favor of the elemental energy of the drives' (Deleuze 1969: 371). For example, concerning the goal that is represented by the final 'becoming' of 'Robinson-Friday,' one can only say (Figure 9.1): *'They' is longer from this world; 'They' now come from the giant sideway ice-planet, Uranus*; *'They' is now Uranian!*

In conclusion, I began my own investigation by asking what use we might have for yet another fable of Robinson Crusoe today. I have argued that the fable is still useful as a cautionary tale concerning the dangers of living in a world without others, especially since everybody (*tout le monde*), in a certain respect, lives on a desert island today. However, I also observed, concerning the original fable of Crusoe, one cannot choose to become a castaway and to live alone on one's own desert island in a world with others, since the 'Other-Structure' is the *a priori* condition of any subject whatsoever. In saying this, I realize that – even before the time of the pandemic –many of my fellow castaways have been experimenting with their own 'desert island sexuality' in an attempt to escape the more oppressive and sad effects of the 'Other-Structure'. I would suggest that the success or failure of your experimentation can be assessed by a simple empirical test that consists of two questions: First question: 'How stable is your own body without organs?' Is it relative smooth and seamless, or is it prone to frequent ruptures, causing you to crash back into the depths of the organic body? In other words, is it smooth and round like a hard-boiled egg, flat like a crepe, or does it always come out looking like scrambled eggs? Second question: 'What role do you assign the 'others' in your immanent plan of Desire?' In other words, are there any real 'others'

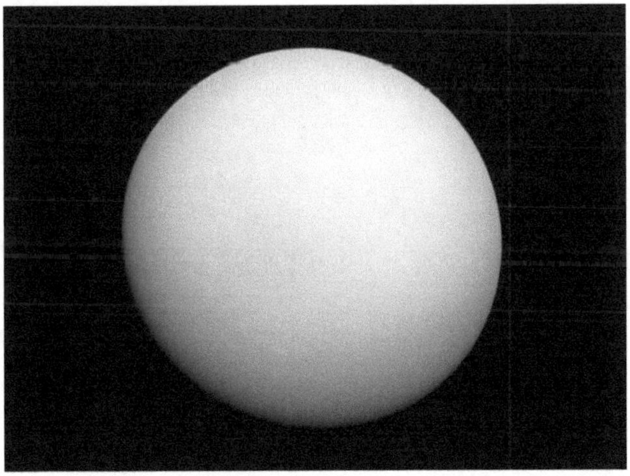

FIGURE 9.1 NASA Voyager 2 photo of the planet Uranus.

Wikipedia Commons at https://commons.wikimedia.org/wiki/File:Uranus2.jpg (accessed 7 May 2021)

living on your desert island, or only the *simulacra* of others (e.g., victims, accomplices, co-conspirators, body-doubles, and body-organs)?

Notes

1 Portions of "Living in a World Without Others" were originally published in *The World Is Gone: Philosophy in Light of the Pandemic* by Gregg Lambert. Published by the University of Minnesota Press, 2021. *The World Is Gone* is licensed under a Creative Commons Attribution-NonCommercial-ShareAlike 4.0 International License (CC BY-NC-SA 4.0). Used by permission.
2 Defoe, 'Serious Observations' in *Robinson Crusoe*, 245.
3 Hereafter, all translation mine.

References

Coetzee, J.M. 1986. *Foe*. London: Penguin Books.
Defoe, Daniel. 1994. *Robinson Crusoe*. New York: W.W. Norton.
Deleuze, Gilles. 1969. *Logique du sens*. Paris: Minuit.
Derrida, Jacques. 2020. *The Beast and the Sovereign*, vol. 2, Translated by Geoffrey Bennington. Chicago: University of Chicago Press.
Heidegger, Martin. 1962. *Being and Time*. New York: Harper & Row.
Levinas, Emmanuel. 2013. *De l'existence à l'existant*. Paris: Vrin.
Tournier, Michel. 1997. *Friday*, Translated by Norman Denny. Baltimore: Johns Hopkins Press.
Woolf, Virginia. 1994. 'Robinson Crusoe' in *Robinson Crusoe*, New York: W.W. Norton, 283–287.

10

THE DITHERING PANDEMIC

David R. Cole

Introduction: A Pandemic, 'the Dithering', and the Anthropocene

Kim Stanley Robinson (2012) characterised the present era (2005–2060) as 'the dithering'. In his fictional framing, and writing retrospectively, historians from the future pinpointed the inability to act according to the science of climate change as 'the dithering'. In this writing, I shall take this notion and apply it to the current circumstances of the COVID-19 pandemic, which have transpired alongside and within the context of what has been termed as 'the Anthropocene' (Crutzen 2002), an age wherein the actions of humans have taken on and represent a 'telluric force'. Hence, we are faced in this epoch (and this chapter) with a conjunction between the pandemic, 'the dithering', and the Anthropocene. The point is not that one has been caused or simply reflects the others, but that within this conjunction are unforeseen and previously unimaginable syntheses, and these are 'productions of the new' (O'Sullivan & Zepke 2008: 1–10) that are determining a period of history which will have far-reaching and profound ramifications in time. To begin to understand these ramifications, I want to make two initial claims, which will be filled out and unpacked throughout the conceptual construction of the essay:

1. One hundred years ago, the First World War, that was closely followed by the Spanish flu pandemic (Barry 2020), gave rise to an unstable period of history that initially saw accelerated economic growth in many countries (the 1920s), followed by the Wall Street crash, the Great Depression, and the rise of highly polarised (left–right) politics, and ultimately the Second World War. We are now in a similar situation. Only the previous détente

DOI: 10.4324/9781003507789-13

of the nuclear standoff prevents a repeat of all-out war (e.g., Weber 1990: 55–65), everything else contained by our circumstances points to a repetition of the events that occurred 100 years ago, with the added pressure of climate change in the Anthropocene – this combined action is here called 'the dithering'.

2. Underneath and within this momentous hundred years 'sine curve' of global history that we are presently living through, there is still the opportunity to think, though I claim that this possibility will be short-lived and is being curtailed in every instance. Once the pandemic subsides, and the superficial fixes and lies with respect to action on climate change that have been 'band-aided' onto the open wound of a warming Earth climate are no longer exposed (cf. Hamilton 2009: 3–15), the invitation to thought will be no more. In other words, the conjunction between the pandemic, 'the dithering', and the Anthropocene simultaneously acts as a disjunction, in that it creates a vacuum wherein thought may travel and pass through the knots and spirals of repeated time to create something new (a third synthesis), and not just repeat the clichés and obvious thought injunctions of every failed project that has brought us to this calamitous point in the first place (Cole 2020: 35–40).

A Philosophy of the Dithering

One hundred years ago, after the First World War and the Spanish flu pandemic, philosophy was not extinguished but had to take on new life and transform itself to survive (e.g., Balakian & Balakian 1986: 56–75). I am arguing that we must do something parallel under the present-day conditions, that I am calling after Robinson as 'the dithering'. In other words, we require 'a philosophy of the dithering' to think – a return to thought. A hundred years ago, philosophy had to change course to explore its underground, the unconscious, nature, death, chaos, weirdness, and previously untouched and negative aspects of human action and thought such as madness. Of course, the impetus to explore such zones had been apparent before (e.g., Newell 2020: 13–60); however, I would like to argue that the combination of World War I and the Spanish flu pandemic functioned as a focusing, as a 'depth-enhancer' for the other side of thought. Today (in 2024), post-pandemic, we could not have imagined the precise circumstances that confront us. Hence, we require tools and concepts whereby we can navigate the conjunction of the pandemic, 'dithering', and the Anthropocene, to find the wormhole through which we can escape its consequences. However, this wormhole is in danger of closure, and it is invisible to most inquiry, as global economic forces and their powers are gathering resources and trying to divert thought along the idiot and suicidal lines that created the deadly conjunction in which we find ourselves trapped.

Language and Affect

Gilles Deleuze (1994a) authored a short essay entitled, 'He Stuttered', in which he paid homage to writers and thinkers who have incorporated 'a stutter' into their writing. Stuttering in this context is not a medical or psychological condition, but a recognition that it is possible to split language apart from the inside, and that great writers can use language in a multidimensional way to open language up upon itself, to reveal what happens within language by language to language, and which is always more complicated than the simple, representational presentation of a written word. Deleuze's (1994a) engagement with the stuttering of written language was consistent throughout his career, and he uses this motif to critique other philosophical approaches such as analytical philosophy and phenomenology, which do not ecognize the power of stuttering and that could be said to underpin *the language of dithering*. For example, in the *Logic of Sense*:

> It is only by breaking open the circle, as in the case of the Möbius strip, by unfolding and untwisting it, that the dimension of sense appears for itself, in its irreducibility, and in its genetic power as it animates an *a priori* internal model of the proposition. (Deleuze 1990: 20)

Deleuze's (1990) concern in the *Logic of Sense* is to unlock sense through nonsense, by deploying, for example, Lewis Carroll's *Alice Through the Looking Glass*, as well as series mathematics and the ancient philosophy of the Stoics (Sellars 2006: 157–164). Underneath and beyond the engagement with sense, propositional language, and the subject of language in the *Logic of Sense* is the notion of schizophrenia that Deleuze would build into a major concept through his joint works with Félix Guattari (1984, 1988). Guattari was a recognized anti-psychiatrist at La Borde Institute outside of Paris and had been a student of Lacan (Martino 2017: 120). He had developed an innovative approach to treating schizophrenia, based on shifting models of consciousness to enable the freeing of schizo energies and thought rather than trapping them in the subject, as might have been the case with psychoanalysis and the analysis of dreams. This method for unlocking the unconscious was developed and ecognize further in Deleuze/Guattari's (1984: 273–383) first joint publication, *Anti-Oedipus*, and was called 'schizoanalysis'. Schizoanalysis primarily depends upon recognizing and acting upon 'the trembling of affect', as Guattari (cf. Cole 2016: 145–152) would call it, and instead of encircling and delimiting such trembling, explores the means and conceptual architecture to understand, preserve, follow, and augment it. For example, in our situation of the COVID-19 pandemic, the point is not to simply entrap, denigrate, or not mention in public the effects of the virus, but to recognize, explicate, and to be moved by its 'trembling affects', here as dithering. As such, the virus is a gateway to a whole new means of affect and expression, and not a dead-end to be eliminated and forgotten at all costs, or simply to be treated with medicine, protocols, or procedures. The truth is that like the Spanish flu one hundred years ago (Barry 2020), we need to find a dithering, non-exterminatory, expressive means to live with the virus, just as we currently live with every other potentially deadly disease that is circulating around the globe. One way to resolve such a problem and paradox is to think of the machine aspects of the pandemic.

Machines

We live in a world that is run by machines. We can understand nature (and our place in it) as a machine (cf. Marshall 2015: 1–52). However, it takes events such as COVID-19, or an economic or natural crisis, for us to realise the functioning of these machines. Now, in the aftermath of the pandemic, we may understand the complexities of the machines in which we live on every inter-related level, from the micro-biological and how the virus attacks our organism to the social, economic, and cultural, and how COVID-19 has transformed these activities, and, ultimately these deliberations can lead to considerations as to cosmic effects and our irrelevant place in the universe. In short, the switching of thought to that of the machine eliminates subjectivity as ego, and belonging to a specific person, or talk of an isolated consciousness and how, in the case of this article, it might relate to dithering and the pandemic (i.e., the dithering within). The dithering is a machine, as it contains and is contained by machine components that relate to the pandemic and the Anthropocene, or how humans have become embroiled in the dynamics of climate change through their actions and drives (e.g., Shove 2010: 277–285) and have at the same time helped to spread a global virus as a pandemic. As such, the dithering machine is part of the change mechanisms that are creating a new world, and yet it is productive of imaginative processes that help to refocus and redistribute the effects of the machine along different lines, as suggested in this quote from Tomkins (1965):

> The skyscraper itself is a kind of machine. The American house is a machine. I saw in my mind's eye all those skyscrapers, those monster buildings, all that magnificent accumulation of human power and vitality, all that uneasiness, as though everyone were living on the edge of a precipice, and I thought how nice it would be to make a little machine there that would be conceived, like Chinese fireworks, in total anarchy and freedom.
>
> *(166)*

As presented in the foregoing quote, the consequent 'dithering machine' does not function perfectly and is not perfectible. In other words, it is full of glitches, repetitions that go nowhere, ghosts (in the machine) (Cole & Hager 2010: 21–35), and it presents the means and resources to inspire counter-intuitive lines of thought and actions. In the world of art, Paul Klee's 'twittering machine' (Shapiro, 1968) suggests a parallel to the dithering machine, as well as Jean Tinguely's useless kinetic machines (Bradley 2018: 193–201). In cinema, Luis Bunuel's (1972) *The Discreet Charm of the Bourgeoisie* creates a dithering machine that re-enacts a group sitting down to dinner and continually being absurdly interrupted. In Pinter's (1961) play *The Birthday Party*, a dithering machine is created out of an innocent celebratory seaside event, and that throws the scenario into internal paralysis and external confusion. Lastly, the writer Henry Green (1946) creates a dithering machine in his novel *Back*, when a returning soldier from World War II called Charley finds that his darling Rose is dead, but he is unable to mourn, as she had been involved with another man whilst he was away, and he falls in love with a different woman, mistakenly believing her to be the dead Rose. In other words, by giving attention to the repetitions and coincidences in forms and events, one may create 'dithering machines' that are mechanisms for understanding how repetitious and contingent situations coincide and diverge along the timelines in our lives. Guattari (2019) used machine structures to destructuralise the unconscious; Deleuze (1994b: 70–129) looked at repetitions of the same to restructure philosophy – in the context of this article, 'the dithering machine' works with respect to the nature of the pandemic, and how it relates to the Anthropocene. At another level of undergirding to the ideas that have been presented, and how the dithering relates to language, affect, and the machine, is the philosophical impulse to think otherwise to prevailing norms, and how that intention can impact on the pandemic as dithering.

Libidinal Materialism

The fundamental problems of the pandemic and the Anthropocene are interrelated and work in combination to separate action from thought as dithering. For example, there are solutions to climate change, whether it be drawdown (Hawken 2017: 1–53), regenerative farming (Toensmeier 2016: 1–123), or switching to renewable energy sources and overall living more ecologically. However, these solutions are not enacted globally, due to poor leadership with little thought of the future, and governments concerned to keep economic growth intact by remaining part of the integrated processes of global capitalism that are intimately connected to fossil fuel production and profit. Such dislocation is what is being termed here as 'the dithering'. Similarly, the pandemic inspires such dithering in that the scientific solutions are well-known, such as physical distancing, good hygiene, mask wearing, and remaining in quarantine if infected. However, these simple acts are not universally followed or enacted, because of the disconnect between thought and action produced by the dithering (e.g., the idea that the pandemic is a conspiracy). To get inside this disconnection and disjunction that we are calling the dithering, we require a philosophy that charts these inner relations, and analyses their disruption and irrevocable dislocation. I would like to suggest that the combined thought of George Bataille and the early Nick Land has the power to investigate such territory. For example:

> … But the copula of terms is no less irritating than the copulation of bodies. And when I scream I AM THE SUN an integral erection results, because the verb to be is the vehicle of amorous frenzy …
>
> *(Bataille 1985: 5)*

This quote from Bataille (1985: 5) demonstrates the type of philosophical investigation necessary to examine the dithering of the pandemic (and Anthropocene). Rather than the verb 'to be' being the object of phenomenological investigation, or the conjunction of terms being part of a rational analytical study, Bataille has combined the study of language with being through a third term, which in this piece he names as 'the solar anus' (Bataille 1985: 5–9). Bataille applied this method to other areas such as anthropology, the study of religion, and economics (Bataille 1988), and in our situation it helps to understand what is happening with respect to the dithering. The dithering is not reasonable, or thought through language or 'Being' alone; rather, the dithering is an (unstable) third term, which is outrageous and absurd but relevant and agentic nonetheless. The 'solar anus' provokes thought about the possible routing of the sun through the anus and is a rendition of what Bataille called 'base materialism' (Noys 1998). Base materialism was an attempt to steer a course away from the idealism of surrealism (Bataille 2018: 87–90), and the structural integrity of Marxism (dialectic materialism) that required a proletariat revolution to function and resulted in the Russian totalitarianism of Stalin. In sum, the base materialism of Bataille was an attempt to create a philosophy that connected all levels of human endeavour to natural processes, and especially brought in 'the other' as a fully embraced aspect of and for material thought, for example:

> It is time to abandon the world of the civilized and its light. It is too late to want to be reasonable and learned, which has led to a life without attractions. Secretly or not, it is necessary to become other, or else cease to be.
>
> *(Bataille 2018: 124)*

The dithering responds to this 'base material other' in that it is the very mechanism and routing for avoidance of the realities which we face today (pandemic/Anthropocene). It is interesting that Bataille (2018: 94) broke with surrealism and Breton because he found the movement too bourgeois and idealistic. Rather, he sought a different path out of the First World War and the Spanish flu pandemic, which charted a deeper and more complex ground, and that had remained unexplored by mainstream intellectual thought. For example, his notion of 'dépense', or useless waste, enables questioning of the creation of capitalist surplus, and the universal utilitarianism that permeates thought then and now (Bataille 1988: 20–32). To introduce dépense as the sovereign act, as the most committed and enthusiastic thing you can do, is to reverse the system of values based on creating surplus value and henceforth products being described as useful. Dépense is giving away what is most valuable, whether it be your life as in sacrificing yourself, or more obliquely as not obeying the economic laws of consumption and accumulation. In the context of this article, dépense responds to one of Bataille's most innovative advocates, Nick Land, when he suggests that "it is the unintelligibility of the world alone that gives it worth" (Land 2011: 167). Land (1992) reformulated Bataille's 'base materialism' as 'libidinal materialism', thus eliminating the distinction between base and superstructure, which held vestiges of a Marxian heritage for Bataille (1988). Rather, libidinal materialism:

> resists a relation of reciprocal transcendence against time and departs from the rigorous passivity of physical substance without recourse to dualistic, idealistic, or theistic conceptuality. It implies a process of mutation which is simultaneously devoid of agency and irreducible to the causal chain.
>
> *(Land 1992: 41)*

Hence, the reformulated Landian libidinal materialism more closely follows natural processes and does not impose the artificial, human designation and separation of base and high as does Bataille (1988). The early Land was adamant to create a philosophy that surgically cut away the last vestiges of human intervention on and as thought and sought power and energy in the natural world that rendered the notion of the human as initiator of thought and subjectivity as trivial. In terms of continental philosophy, the early Land (2011) rigorously attacked any philosophy that sought refuge in human intelligence, the transcendental 'I', or any recourse to a soul. Rather, we travel (with Land) in a soulless universe with no human subject to guide and/or constrain us. All that exists are abstract force diagrams, of which we are a small part, propelled along by energy, here called libido, though such impetus does not imply the sole or privileged reserve of human sexuality. In these terms, the dithering is an example of the ways in which these force diagrams have come together and diverge through this era in history. In other words, according to libidinal materialism, the dithering is compositional and Dionysian in the way that it reveals aspects of the unconscious through its movements and effects on the current situation. Such compositionality makes plain, for example, how difficult it is to change aspects of the current situation (e.g., climate change/pandemic infection), because contemporary global capitalism, which is driving both processes, is fully able to participate as and through libidinal materialism in its continued augmentation (as capitalism–global warming–pandemic). In contrast, well-meaning, earnest, and correct pro-environmental and health schemes fail precisely because they do not participate at the level of libidinal materialism, which has:

> the power to conserve, transmit, circulate, and enhance compositions, the power that is assimilated in the marking, reserving, and appropriating of compositions, and the power released in the disinhibition, dissipation, and Dionysian unleashing of compositions ...
>
> *(Land 1992: 44)*

Simulacrum

Lastly, in term of constructing a philosophy of the dithering, it is worth exploring the notion of the simulacrum as the dithering and a vital, linking concept, as it appears in Klossowski, Deleuze, and Baudrillard (Smith 2005: 100–120). The simulacrum was taken up and used in quite separate ways by each author. Deleuze (1994b: 278) deployed the simulacrum for philosophical reasons, to differentiate his ideas from the Platonic copy and the resultant idealism; Baudrillard (1983: 67–75) used the simulacrum to explain the complex, imagistic, and semiotic mechanisms of capitalist production, reproduction, and the capturing of the self through marketing and the profit margin; Klossowski (2017: 51–73) took the notion of the simulacrum to help found the body in the eternal return. One could argue that Klossowski's ideas are an anathema to the ways in which body may be enslaved, copied, and divided from the mind due to Platonic mind/body dualism, or in the Christian rendition of the soul, which alone can go to heaven. Further, Klossowski's notion of the body functions outside of capitalist exchange, as it is a simulacrum of the 'thought-destiny' entailed by the eternal recurrence. Hence, as a frozen concept, entirely 'choiceless' in the repetitions of time, and as being a shaky, uncertain part of the metaphysics of nihilism and belief in nothingness that one may derive from the eternal return, the dithering (as simulacrum) does not take part in the possession of the body as laid out by the commercialisation of the present moment, as Klossowski (2017) explained in *Living Currency*:

> As soon as the bodily presence of the industrial slave is absolutely included in figuring the appraisable yield of what he or she can produce (their physiognomy being inseparable from their work), it is specious to draw a distinction between a person and their activity.

> Bodily presence is already a commodity, independent of and over and above the commodity itself that such presence contributes to producing. And now, industrial slaves must either establish a strict relationship between their bodily presence and the money it brings in, or replace the function of money, and be money themselves: simultaneously the equivalent of wealth, and wealth itself.
>
> *(2017: 6)*

As such, the simulacrum of the dithering has no body and does not take part in the possession of the body or in the industrial exchange as suggested by Klossowski (2017: 10). According to Klossowski, a simulacrum is a willed re-creation of a phantasm in a literary, pictorial, or plastic form, which simulates the invisible agitation of the mind. In both senses, the simulacrum is related to myth as far as myth is the narrative manifestation of unconscious, primordial forces (Nietzsche 1974: 12). Therefore, the unconscious is opened in the way the simulacrum works, simultaneously on the personal and social/machine levels, and includes the tendency to expunge or destroy trivial, moralistic, and interpretive views of the unconscious. Hence, the simulacrum as the dithering acts as part of the eternal recurrence, and this 'situatedness' recreates an agonistic attitude to the current moment, as has been expressed through various philosophies such as those of Nietzsche (1974), Deleuze (1994a, 1994b), Guattari (2012), Bataille (1988), or Land (1992). Further, Klossowski's simulacrum (and hence the dithering) is riven through with the ideas of the Marquis de Sade, which again takes us away from the present moment and the multitude of occasions and voices through which moralistic, social, and personal forces can intervene on our thoughts to sublimate and distract from the reality in which we live. Klossowski (2017: 23) suggests that it takes a similar force as the Marquis de Sade to question the prevailing morals and norms in his time to understand how the simulacrum works as the dithering to take us out of the bodily, imagistic, and spectacular loops that trap us today:

> Abolishing property ownership over one's own body and over the body of others is an operation inherent in the pervert's imagination; he inhabits the bodies of others as if they were his own, and thus attributes his own to others. This means that his own body itself comes back to him as a domain of fantasy; thus, it becomes merely the equivalent of the fantasy – it is its **simulacrum**.
>
> *(Klossowski 2017: 24)*

It is unclear whether Klossowski (2017) is suggesting that we necessarily become à la Sade to escape the evacuation of the self through bodily exchange as executed in capitalism, or if he is intending that we augment the processes already apparent in commercial exchange as a mode of accelerationism (Sellar & Cole 2017). What is clear is that Klossowski is reconfiguring the simulacrum in terms of a positive artistic and philosophical project – through which one might avoid being captured by image-exchange under capitalism and reconfigure the unconscious in a non-interpretative manner to resist and disrupt the action of capital on how and what we imagine and dream. On these terms, the dithering relates to what the body can do and is subject to. The dithering is deliberately held at the edge of the imagination, and that resists mainstream, normative interpretation. The dithering as a simulacrum works immanently, as an intervention about what can be thought and desired. In this sense, the dithering is not simply additive or negatory in terms of how it fits in with the complex regimes of exchange that we experience through capitalism. In sum, the dithering as a simulacrum is a path through the recurrences of time, which leads us to another place through image, and away from the incessant chatter of the commerciality of now.

White Noise for Postmedia

In sum, the philosophy of the dithering that has been constructed in this chapter is a mode of introducing white noise, or as important background effects that help to highlight the ways in which the pandemic relates to the Anthropocene in the contemporary era (Figure 10.1), and how to escape them. White noise is transmissible through Guattari's conception of postmedia (1990), or the notion that 'corpuscles of communication' may be effective in disrupting and rerouting the mainstream, commercial, bland, stupefying modes in which the media is currently deployed. Figure 10.1 acts as a blueprint and signpost for the ways in which this white noise for postmedia may be constructed for the dithering:

Key to understanding how this plan for introducing white noise into a postmedia landscape works is thinking through one of Guattari's primary concerns, that of social change. The dithering encapsulates the inability to act on scientific fact, such as that of global warming, or how human effects are changing the climate in the Anthropocene (Ruddiman 2013: 60). The dithering is the contingency at this base of indecision and may be understood philosophically through stuttering, affect, machines, libidinal materialism, and the simulacrum. Guattari (1990) envisaged that subjectivity could be changed through the micro appropriation of media that he called postmedia, which in his day revolved around radio and television, but now has morphed dramatically through the internet and social media. The point is that the dithering introduces a mark of contingency into the plan for social change that Guattari (1990) dreamed of, and that acts as a defence against the multiple ways in which any plan to change society may be hijacked and derailed by the forces of global capitalism. The white noise of the dithering needs to be sustained

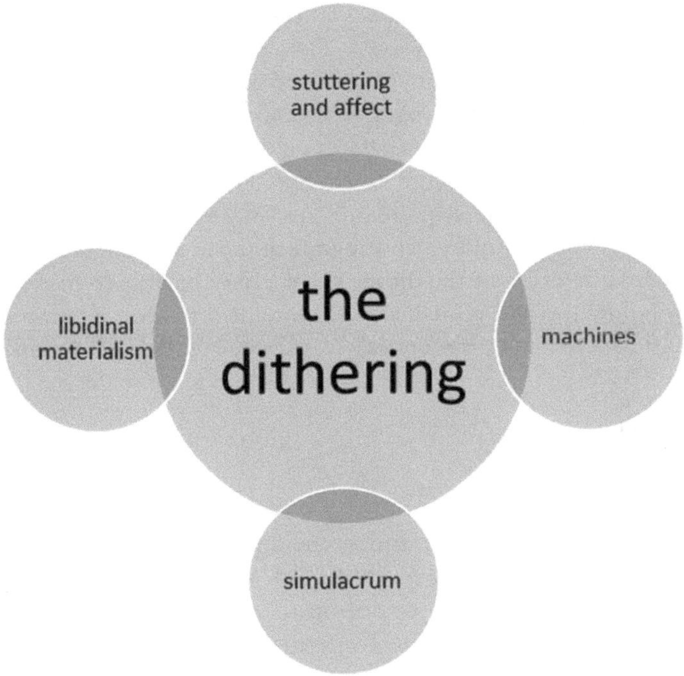

FIGURE 10.1 'The dithering' and its component influences.

and powerful enough not to be extinguished by the barrage of strategies, communications, and diversions that will be thrown at it by the mainstream capitalism majority. As such, the postmedia is a device or apparatus whereby the white noise of the dithering is not dismissed or ignored as so much interference or background but augmented and operationalised. This logic of dithering inter-relationships adds complexity to societal change, and at the same time encourages understanding of the present moment (as the dithering), and that introduces and deploys the processes of meta-modelling as Guattari (Cole 2016) described them. These processes of meta-modelling may be understood by the cybernetic statement:

> Planning society is impossible because the elaboration and implementation of plans always must operate as processes within the societal system. Trying to plan the society would create a state in which planning and other forms of behaviour exist side by side and react on each other. Planners may use a description of the system; they may introduce a simplified version of the complexity of the system into the system. But this will only produce a hypercomplex system which contains within itself a description of its own complexity.
>
> *(Luhmann 1990: 137)*

Guattari's (2012) meta-modelling is a method to understand how the hypercomplexity of social planning works. This is because society is a metamorphic system, with plans within plans, and lines of escape and digression wrought into its very functioning and thought. Guattari's concepts work to establish a definite link between the unconscious and how society works, even during a pandemic and climate change. Pointedly, the circumstances in which we find ourselves post pandemic are in need of an exit route, and at least Guattari (1990) supplies a routing mechanism to feed into society. If we can hear the white noise of the dithering, we may be able to move towards a postmedia landscape and reinvent and create new modes of communication, thinking, and society (as cybernetics).

Conclusion(s)

Thinking through the Dithering

Thinking is being torn apart by and as the dithering; yet this paper, which is about the dithering, and how to think during a pandemic (and post pandemic), has its focus on this very notion of separation and merging, or the oscillation happening due to the dithering. The dithering is not solely a human matter but part of a thought-destiny contained and functioning as the contemporary moment, and how circumstances such as the pandemic and Anthropocene are routing and rerouting thought in ways that act as dislocation between what we know, what we think, and what we do (cf. Crist 2019: 103–16). It is the contention of this paper that philosophy is still possible in the situation of a pandemic, post pandemic, and the Anthropocene, yet only if the escape route as suggested previously is created, that is, as stuttering, affect, machines, libidinal materialism, and simulacrum. The combined effects of this philosophy of the dithering, which is designed to be reformulated as white noise to be broadcast through Guattari's (1990) postmedia, stipulates micro growths or self-reciprocating blooms in communication, thought, and action. Guattari's strategic fluidity between nodes of thought and becoming is meant to avoid detection and use by top-down capitalist or corporate interests, which would seek to coopt and exploit these growths. As such, the dithering as theorised previously and to be broadcast through the postmedia conforms to Adorno's (2007) statement with respect to how industrial society is simultaneously our hope and undoing:

> There is a universal feeling, a universal fear, that our progress in controlling nature may increasingly help to weave the very calamity it is supposed to protect us from.
>
> *(2007: 67)*

References

Adorno, T.W. 2007. *Negative Dialectics*. Translated by E.B. Ashton. Continuum.

Balakian, A. and Balakian, A.E. 1986. *Surrealism: The Road to the Absolute*. Chicago and London: University of Chicago Press.

Barry, J.M. 2020. *The Great Influenza: The Story of the Deadliest Pandemic in History*. UK: Penguin.

Bataille, G. 1985. *Visions of Excess: Selected Writings, 1927–1939* in A. Stoekl (ed.), Translated by A. Stoekl, C.R. Lovitt & D.M. Leslie. Minneapolis: University of Minnesota Press.

Bataille, G. 1988. *The Accursed Share* (Vol. 1), Translated by R Hurley. New York: Zone Books.

Bataille, G. 2018. *Sacred Conspiracy: The Internal Papers of the Secret Society of Acephale and Lecturers to the College of Sociology*. London: Atlas Press.

Baudrillard, J. 1983. *Simulacra and Simulations*. Translated by P. Foss, P. Patton, & P. Beitchman. New York: Semiotext(e).

Bradley, J.P. 2018. The delirious abstract machines of Jean Tinguely, in P. Maccormack & C. Gardner (eds.), *Ecosophical Aesthetics: Art, Ethics and Ecology with Guattari*, 193–217. London: Bloomsbury.

Bunuel, L. (Dir). 1972. *The Discreet Charm of the Bourgeoisie* [film]. 20th Century Fox.

Cole, D.R. 2016. Unearthing the forces of globalisation in educational research through Guattari's cartographic method, in D.R. Cole & C. Woodrow (eds.), *Super Dimensions in Globalisation and Education*. 145–159. Singapore: Springer.

Cole, D.R. 2020. Learning to think in the Anthropocene: What Can Deleuze-Guattari teach us? in K. Maiti & S. Chakraborty(eds.), *Global Perspectives on Eco-Aesthetics and Eco-Ethics: A Green Critique*, 31–47. Maryland: Lexington Books.

Cole, D.R., & P. Hager. 2010. Learning-practice: The ghosts in the education machine. *Education Inquiry*, *1*(1): 21–40.

Crist, E. 2019. *Abundant Earth: Toward an Ecological Civilization*. Chicago: University of Chicago Press.

Crutzen, P.J. 2002. Geology of mankind. *Nature*, 415, 23.

Deleuze, G. 1990. *The Logic of Sense*. C.V. Boundas (ed.), Translated by M. Lester. London: The Athlone Press.

Deleuze, Gilles. 1994a. He stuttered, in C.V. Boundas & D. Olkowski (eds.), *The Theatre of Philosophy*, 24–31. London: Routledge.

Deleuze, Gilles. 1994b. *Difference & Repetition*. Translated by Paul Patton. New York: Columbia University Press.

Deleuze, Gilles and Felix Guattari. 1984. *Anti-Oedipus: Capitalism & Schizophrenia*. Translated by R. Hurley, M. Steen, & H.R. Lane. New York: The Athlone Press.

Deleuze, Gilles and Felix Guattari. 1988. *A Thousand Plateaus: Capitalism and Schizophrenia II*. Translated by Brian Massumi. London: The Athlone Press.

Green, H. 1946. *Back*. London: Hogarth Press.

Guattari, Felix. 1990. Towards a post media era. Translated by A. Sebti & C. Apprich. *Chimères*, 28.

Guattari, Felix. 2012. *Schizoanalytic cartographies*. Translated by A. Goffey. London: Bloomsbury.

Guattari, Felix. 2019. Machine and structure. *Novoe Literaturnoe Obozrenie*, 158, 70–78.

Hamilton, C. 2009. Is it too late to prevent catastrophic climate change? in *Lecture to a Meeting of the Royal Society of the Arts, Sydney* (Vol. 21). Metro DC Committee of Correspondence for Democracy and Socialism (CCDS): https://www.redandgreen.org/Climate_Change/rsa_lecture-1.pdf

Hawken, P. 2017. *Drawdown: The Most Comprehensive Plan Ever Proposed to Reverse Global Warming*. UK: Penguin.

Klossowski, P. 2017. *Living Currency*. Translated by & (eds) V.W. Cisney, N. Morar & D.W. Smith. London: Bloomsbury.

Land, Nick. 1992. *The Thirst for Annihilation*. London: Routledge.

Land, Nick. 2011. *Fanged Noumena: Collected Writings 1987–2007*. Cambridge: MIT Press.

Luhmann, N. 1990. *Essays on Self-Reference*. New York: Columbia University Press.

Marshall, P. 2015. *Nature's Web: Rethinking Our Place on Earth: Rethinking Our Place on Earth*. London: Routledge.

Martino, B.L. 2017. *The Living Inside: Listening to Madness with Félix Guattari* [Doctoral dissertation]. State University of New York at Stony Brook.

Newell, J. 2020. *A Century of Weird Fiction, 1832–1937: Disgust, Metaphysics and the Aesthetics of Cosmic Horror*. Cardiff, UK: University of Wales Press.

Nietzsche, F. 1974. *The Gay Science: with a prelude in rhymes and an appendix of songs*. Translated by W. Kaufmann. New York: Vintage Books.

Noys, B. 1998. Georges Bataille's base materialism. *Journal for Cultural Research*, 2(4), 499–517.

O'Sullivan, Simon and Stephen Zepke (eds.). 2008. *Deleuze, Guattari and the Production of the New*. London: Bloomsbury.

Pinter, H. 1961. *The Birthday Party, and The Room: Two Plays* (Vol. 315). Grove Press.

Robinson, K.S. 2012. *2312*. Orbit books.

Ruddiman, W.F. 2013. The anthropocene. *Annual Review of Earth and Planetary Sciences*, 41, 45–68.

Sellar, S. and David R. Cole. 2017. 'Accelerationism: A timely provocation for the critical sociology of education. *British Journal of Sociology of Education*, *38*(1), 38–48.

Sellars, J. 2006. 'An ethics of the event: Deleuze's stoicism. *Angelaki: Journal of the Theoretical Humanities*, *11*(3), 157–171.

Shapiro, M.L. 1968. Klee's Twittering Machine. *The Art Bulletin*, *50*(1), 67–69.

Shove, E. 2010. 'Social theory and climate change. *Theory, Culture & Society*, *27*(2–3), 277–288.

Smith, D.W. 2005. 'The concept of the simulacrum: Deleuze and the overturning of Platonism. *Continental Philosophy Review*, *38*(1–2), 89–123.

Toensmeier, E. 2016. *The Carbon Farming Solution: A Global Toolkit of Perennial Crops and Regenerative Agriculture Practices for Climate Change Mitigation and Food Security*. Vermont: Chelsea Green Publishing.

Tomkins, C. 1965. *The Bride and the Bachelors: Five Masters of the Avant-Garde*. New York: Viking Press.

Weber, S. 1990. Realism, Detente, and Nuclear Weapons. *International Organization*, *44*(1), 55–82. http://www.jstor.org/stable/2706809

11

QUARANTINE OR FEAST?

Hospitality and the State of Plague

Janell Watson

Introduction

The Covid-19 pandemic caused by the SARS-CoV-2 virus has been met with two divergent social responses. The first, which I label 'quarantine', includes masking, social distancing, and self-isolating at home behind closed doors. The second, which I label 'feast', includes gathering together, largely unmasked, in restaurants, bars, churches, entertainment venues, or private homes opened up to others. To quarantine is to separate from others in the interest of public health in order to protect human life from the virus. To feast is to commune with others in the interests of social and economic exchange in order to enjoy life despite the virus. These two social responses to life during a pandemic – quarantine or feast – can be described in terms of the ancient laws of hospitality, as explicated by Michel Serres and Jacques Derrida, who note the lexical and historical proximity of *hospitality* to *hostility*. In Greek, *xenos* 'designates the foreigner, but it also designates the guest', an outsider invited inside. In Latin, *hostis* means both host and enemy. Similarly, the French word *hôte* means both host and guest (Serres 2015a: 162; Derrida and Dufourmantelle 2000: 19, 41, 43, 45). The act of hospitality blurs the stranger–guest distinction, transforming the potentially hostile stranger into a welcomed guest. Derrida's coinage 'hostipality' combines hospitality with hostility, highlighting this crossing of the outside–inside boundary (Derrida 2000).

Virology, the scientific response to viruses, also 'uses the vocabulary of the host' (Serres 1982: 193). A virus is a parasite whose survival depends on entering a living host. In French and English, the word *parasite* designates both a biological entity that lives off another organism and also an unwelcome guest,

DOI: 10.4324/9781003507789-14

especially one who arrives uninvited and overstays their welcome. Like an uninvited guest at a feast, the SARS-CoV-2 virus enters the host from the outside, a foreign body feasting on its hospitable host. Invading then replicating within the host body, the virus proves to be a hostile guest. The propensity of the virus to move from one host to another transforms the latter into a potentially dangerous guest – an enemy harbouring an enemy. Roberto Esposito combines the vocabulary of virology with that of political philosophy in creating the notion of biopolitical immunity. The immune system, of a biological or social body, launches a 'violent defense' against intruders, attacking anything perceived as 'foreign' (Esposito 2011: 17). An overly zealous immune response threatens the social bonds of the community. Should it come as a surprise that quarantine measures have been met with hostility?

To quarantine is to refuse social hospitality so as to avoid the risk of hosting a guest whom the biological virus has transformed into an enemy. To feast is to give or receive hospitably, maintaining social relations and economic well-being, despite the risk of letting in the uninvited biological parasite. Are economic health and social health less important than biological health? Different populations and governments have responded differently to the threat of biological intrusion. Some advocate imposing a quarantine in an effort to save lives, while others argue that it is more important to live life by feasting. States and their populations struggle with the question of hospitality, in a world that has grown dependent on a large hospitality industry that thrives on travel and consumption – a global feast.[1] The global networks of the feast economy serve as viral vectors, as exemplified by the now iconic *Diamond Princess* cruise ship. Quarantine shut down the feast economy, resulting in layoffs and business closures that widened the already deep divide between those who enjoy the feasts and those who serve them.

Covid-19 was declared a global pandemic during a US presidential election that has been repeatedly described as particularly divisive. These divergent behaviours, quarantining and feasting, were mapped onto the red–blue political divide, the Republican candidate hosting large in-person rallies and gatherings at the White House, while the Democrat candidate campaigned from the family basement in Delaware, hosting only socially distanced online or drive-in events. Republicans feasted while Democrats quarantined. The quarantine party narrowly defeated the feasting party in the November 2020 election, but no nationwide masking mandate has been imposed in the US. Rules and regulations were left to local governments who followed, or not, national recommendations. The result was a mixture of quarantining and masking. Internationally, many nations masked and quarantined, while others remained largely open, and a great many more alternated between quarantine and feast. Alberto Toscano points out the contradictions of 'the pandemic state': right-wing authoritarians like Trump and Bolsonaro opposed 'the militarisation of everyday life', while leftists and liberals advocated 'a greater use of the state's repressive and juridical resources to secure collective well-being' (2020: 14; see also Žižek 2020: 73–77, 91–93).

The question of state-mandated quarantine measures emerged as a point of debate among European philosophers (Toscano 2020; Peters 2020; Castrillón and Marchevsky 2021). In February 2020, just as talk of a pandemic emerged in the world news, Giorgio Agamben denounced quarantine as the imposition of the 'state of exception' which justifies state-mandated restrictions on movement and daily life. He cites Michel Foucault's writings on quarantine as a paradigm of modern state control by means of separation and data collection (Agamben 2020). Alain Badiou countered that there is nothing exceptional or new about epidemics or pandemics, which have always plagued humans and remain a threat to this day. Badiou unequivocally advocates state-imposed quarantine, claiming that 'Reason' (his capitalization and quotation marks) dictates this inhospitable response (Badiou 2020).

I myself practice quarantine and continue avoiding collective feasts even after being vaccinated but, as a reader of Serres, I question Badiou's claim to 'Reason'. I am not asking whether or not Serres (who died in 2019, before the present pandemic) would have advocated quarantine or feast, but instead explore his quest for a more hospitable reason, as he seeks wisdom in ancient Roman ritual feasts, denounces the false gods of today's feast economy, and advocates for a politics of care predicated on absolute hospitality.

State of Uncertainty

Characterising the Covid-19 pandemic as an unexceptional situation, Badiou offers what he calls a 'Cartesian' response that brings together 'some simple ideas'. The complexity of an epidemic, he says, results from the intersection of two determinations, a natural determination and a social one. To analyse the complexities of the current pandemic, he says, 'one must grasp the points at which the two determinations intersect and draw the consequences'. He references the then-prevailing hypothesis that the first human case of Covid-19 originated at a live animal market in Wuhan, China. Naturally determined, the current pandemic was caused by a virus that spread from animals to humans at a local market. Socially determined, the disease grew into pandemic as humans transported the virus via the global marketplace of goods and services. The local (animal market) intersects the global (world economy) at the same point where the natural intersects the social (Badiou 2020).

Claiming 'Reason', Badiou defends political states – including France – that impose quarantine measures in order to stop the further spread of the natural virus along social networks. Quarantine, he says,

> is an entirely *logical consequence* of the situation, the aim of which is to stifle the epidemic – to win the war, to borrow once again Macron's

> metaphor – with the greatest *certainty* possible, while remaining within the established social order. This is no laughing matter, it is a *necessity* imposed by the diffusion of a lethal process that intersects nature (whence the preeminent role of scientists in the matter) and the social order (whence the authoritarian intervention, and it couldn't be otherwise, of the state).
>
> *(Badiou 2020: my emphasis)*

Badiou chooses quarantine over feast, claiming that 'certainty' and logical 'necessity' dictate an 'authoritarian intervention' on the part of the state in its 'war' against the epidemic. Suggesting that quarantine is not incompatible with maintaining 'the established social order', he dismisses Agamben's claim that quarantine amounts to the imposition of a state of exception that will destroy the democratic social order of a state like Italy. To borrow Toscano's framework for evaluating state responses to the Covid-19 pandemic, Agamben 'fears' the state for its power to oppress, while Badiou 'desires' the state for its power to protect (Toscano 2020: 3). Badiou fears the virus more than he fears the state, and so desires state-imposed quarantine. Thus formulated, it seems to me that Badiou chooses quarantine on the basis of a risk calculation, undertaking a calculus of probabilities as to which option presents the greatest threat to living life, the virus or the state. He has not simply followed a Cartesian chain of logical deduction but has rather made a wager in the spirit of Leibniz and Pascal.

Serres contrasts the simple Cartesian chain of reason against the complex networks of determination woven by Leibniz (Serres 1968b: 113–153; 1983: 17–18, 24–28). He associates claims to Cartesian reason with the pursuit of power by means of a reductionist elimination of uncertainty, which amounts to a philosophical authoritarianism. 'The stable chain of the rationalists only expresses, I think, their desire of domination' writes Serres, who frequently denounces Descartes's call for the human mastery and possession of nature (see for example 1983: 21; 1995b: 33–34; 1997: 72). While Badiou is of course justified in stating with certainty that the present pandemic is caused by the SARS-CoV-2 virus, any 'authoritarian intervention' on the part of a state is a political choice, even if it is justified by scientific evidence. I am not questioning Badiou's advocacy of quarantine (which is my own position as well), but rather his claim to reason, necessity, and certitude. Science itself remains uncertain about many aspects of the nature of the virus and its interaction with its hosts' cells, and social science offers even less certitude about how to predict or manage human social behaviour.

Modern science in fact embraces uncertainty, argues Serres. It may be tempting to describe today's maskers and vaxxers as rationalists acting out of scientific certitude, and the anti-maskers and anti-vaxxers as irrationally doubtful of science, but things are not so simple. Contemporary science finds uncertainty in the universe itself, as expressed by Gödel's incompleteness theorem, Heisenberg's uncertainty principle, and chaos theory. As Serres puts it, 'the history of our science continually augments the same retreating movement from every position of certainty and puts them in doubt. ... the universe, contingent, evolves contingently, functions according to contingent laws and constants having contingent values' (Serres 2020: 36). Science no longer describes the universe as a clock or solar system with predictable movements, but presents it as more like a weather system, especially at the molecular scales of molecules and cells (Serres 1978: 9–13). Like the weather forecast, the spread of viruses can be calculated only on the basis of incomplete data and predicted only in terms of limits, likelihood, and probability, given viruses' ability to multiply and mutate, resulting in varying degrees of infectiousness and lethality. The contingencies of viral propagation and mutation intersect with the unpredictable behaviours of human or animal hosts. To be clear, there is nothing social about the virus, a primordial piece of nature. 'Suddenly the plague has a virus for its cause, a virus having few relations to our [human] relations', writes Serres (2015a: 175). Modern scientific knowledge of the virus does nothing to solve problems of social relations. Scientists must pay attention to social relations. Politicians must pay attention to science. Philosophers must heed to complexities of their intersection.

In pursuit of Cartesian reason, Badiou explicitly excludes human culture from consideration, lamenting the attention that journalists and other intellectuals are paying to 'those sad effects – mysticism, fabulation, prayer, prophecy and malediction – that were customary in the Middle Ages when plague swept the land' (2020). In stark contrast, Serres, following Leibniz, seeks reason and logic in ritual, myth, and legend. He notes that while Descartes only pays attention to clarity, Leibniz finds reason in the shadows and confusion, and thus welcomes all content, fact or fiction, even the most obscure, with a 'generous hospitality as opposed to Cartesian interdictions'. While Descartes excludes, closing the door to potential sources of knowledge, Leibniz hospitably opens up to all sources, finding flashes of reason in narratives considered 'sterile', 'curious', 'extravagant', or 'obscure', including the works of scholastics, poets, novelists, historians, grammarians, or artisans (Serres 1968a: 119). Leibniz arrives at certitude only after passing through initial obscurity.

Following the Leibnizian example, Serres seeks truths in sources such as Livy's *History of Rome*, which includes legends and myths alongside historical facts. As Serres puts it, describing inhospitable Cartesian exclusion, 'A certain rationalism of old enjoyed eliminating, filtering out the multiple and confusion; it held a little less than a third of what it called the truth' (2015a: 5). Despite their ignorance of modern virology, the Romans understood a thing or two about plague, reasons Serres. Historian Samuel K. Cohn, Jr. also turns to Livy, among other historical and non-historical sources, in order to understand recent pandemics like swine flu and AIDS. Serres explores the same references to ancient Roman plagues in order to understand the emergence of the modern state, which coalesces out of unruly populations, operating as if according to the laws of chaos. He claims that in the realm of politics and the social order, 'nothing much has changed' since the time of the Roman kings (90–91).

'Might as Well Open Our Doors'

Seeking truths in the shadowy legends of human culture, Serres describes a series of ancient Roman feasts offered in response to the state of uncertainty brought about by fear of plague. According to Livy, 'in order to ward off the plague', Rome held these ritual banquets, called *lectisternia*, in public as well as in private. Statues of gods presided at the public feasts. Friends and enemies alike were welcomed to the table. 'During the feast, in the entire city the doors of the houses open ... Those known and those unknown are received; foreigners, even enemies become guests' (Serres 2015a: 161). Hospitality is offered, even to guests who may prove to be hostile.

> General hostility is close, infinitely close to general hospitality. In our ignorance of who is who, friend or hostile, including ourselves, we might as well open the doors wide. Might as well open our doors when we know that the doors no longer protect us.
>
> *(173)*

Since we do not know who or what may carry the enemy pestilence, we might as well feast. Thus Rome responded to uncertainty by hosting banquets.

The *lectisternia* could of course be dismissed as a pre-scientific response to a situation that modern medicine explains by germ theory, but their social role remains relevant. The Romans attributed plague to many causes, says historian Cohn in *Epidemics: Hate and Compassion from the Plague of Athens to AIDS*, not only to the gods' anger at human actions, but also and indeed more frequently to 'natural causes' such as climate fluctuations, miasmas, or overcrowding. Even though the Romans acknowledged crowding as a cause of plague, their *lectisternia* hospitably gathered strangers and foreigners (Cohn 2018: 8–31, 35–43). Serres confesses to not knowing whether any given plague that Livy mentions was a real epidemic or a social crisis. 'I mean that if the history were reporting a recent event, we would be clear about said disease', says Serres. 'But here, the same discourse – the *narrative of uncertainty* in which hospitality can abruptly turn to hostility ... is valid whether it's a question of a social crisis or ... an authentic epidemic. The words say this equivalence', the word *hostis* which can mean both guest and enemy, and the word *hôte* which can mean host or guest (2015a: 172; my emphasis). Whether an ancient plague was an epidemic in the modern scientific sense or merely a social crisis, the narrative of uncertainty prevails.

Opening the doors and inviting everyone to the feast is the opposite of quarantine, which mandates closed doors. Rather than mandating quarantine, Rome hosted feasts. Serres studies Livy in search of the foundations of the modern state. 'The modern state, with its monopoly of power, is a plague state', writes Toscano (2020: 7). He notes that the Covid-19 pandemic highlights an ambivalence toward the state on both the left and the right, a simultaneous 'desire for the state and hatred of government' (16). It is possible to simultaneously desire that the state protect the health of its people, as well as to fear that the hated state will violate privacy and restrict personal freedom. He notes that the famous illustration of Hobbes's *Leviathan* includes a depiction of the plague state. The sovereign head atop the social body gazes on a walled city that is empty except for some soldiers and two plague doctors wearing birdlike masks. 'War and epidemics are the context for the incorporation of now-powerless subjects into the sovereign, as well as for their seclusion in their homes in times of strife and contagion', comments Toscano (6–7). *Leviathan* thus includes both war and plague in its classic organic model of the modern state.

Serres likewise evokes Hobbes in his discussion of plague, but he overlays the organic model of the social body with a mathematical-physical model of the social collective, conceptualised as a set of elements. Serres therefore uses the term 'state' not only in its political sense but also in the sense of systems theory, to describe the order or disorder of the elements in the set. In the physical sciences, a system undergoes phase changes from one state to another, such as when a set of molecules transitions from a solid state to a gaseous state to a liquid state, or from a state of equilibrium to a turbulent state. Serres warns against too easily importing models from the so-called hard sciences into the social sciences, and yet he marvels at how often social systems behave like physical systems. Hobbes's 'state of nature', or the war of all against all, is a disorderly state of generalised hostility, in which everyone is everyone else's enemy, says Serres. The latter in turn describes the 'state of war' as an orderly state of organised hostility directed toward a clearly defined enemy (1997: 83, 119; 2015a: 207–210).

Serres describes the state of plague as an uncertain relation between hostility and hospitality, muddling the friend–enemy distinction. Unlike war, which organises social collectives into camps, clearly delineating friend from enemy, the plague disorganises the social body by making it impossible to identify the invisible enemy, whether the pestilence is attributed to angry gods, miasma, or microbe. Serres therefore characterises the state of plague as 'the equivalence of hostility and hospitality'. Under the state of plague, 'Everyone is no longer the enemy of everyone else; everyone is rather their plague'; this is because 'No one knows who carries the plague, who gives it, who receives it'. To live in a state of plague is to exist in a state of uncertainty. In the state of war, 'The enemy is the enemy ... he is recognised, ordered, foreseeable. It's easy to be wary of him'. In contrast, 'When everyone is the plague of everyone else, all order has vanished, all foreseeability is erased'. Plague is an unpredictable state and thus, suggests Serres, provides an excellent model of 'the relation of uncertainty' that pervades the natural domain of science as well as the social domain of culture (2015a: 164, 169).

Calculating the Leviathan

Unconditional hospitality brings everyone together, mixing friends with enemies, known and unknown. Contemplating the social mixture that results from open hospitality, Serres mixes methods, combining a rustic recipe with political theory and mathematics, bringing together 'a wide variety of scholarly specialities'. He imagines an amalgamation of guests feasting on a Roman dish that mixes fruit, vegetables, and meats, each element remaining discernible. Nothing is excluded; all people and all food groups are welcome. In mathematical language, these heterogeneous mixtures of disparate elements form 'non-standard multiplicities' that exist in a 'non-standardized state' (2015a: 169, 179). Serres is evoking non-standard analysis, a branch of calculus that allows for the infinitesimals that standard calculus excludes. Leibniz found infinitesimals useful, even 'magic', for solving practical problems, but they later fell out of favour because they leave behind paradoxes and nonsensical equations that most mathematicians prefer to ignore. Standard calculus instead relies on approximations that work just fine, even though the infinitesimal approach is arguably more rigorous, if inexact. Abraham Robinson returned to infinitesimals in the 1960s, developing a non-standard analysis that supplied proofs in support of Leibniz's practical success with infinity (Strogatz 2019: 202–209; Robinson 1996). Can the feast, as non-standard multiplicity, serve as a model for a political state that is less exclusionary and more welcoming? This is the question Serres poses in comparing the state of war – the only state Hobbes knows, he says – to the state of plague.

Hobbes anticipates standard calculus, argues Serres, because war and the Leviathan produce standard states, standardising the non-standard multiplicities, eliminating their 'abundance of differences' (2015a: 169).[2] Standard calculus, that powerful mathematical tool that makes our technological age of information possible, operates by dividing a complex problem, like measuring a curved area or volume, into simpler parts that resemble each other. Differentiation divides a continuous curved area into infinitely many small rectangular slices or straight-sided volumes, whose dimensions can be calculated using simple formulas.[3] Integration puts the simplified parts back together again, reintegrating them into a sum – the area or volume of the curved shape (Strogatz 2019: xv, 89, 216–218). The Leviathan relies on this same operation in order to constitute the social body of the modern state, argues Serres. 'A global system can be decomposed into very little local individuals; it's always easy to trace a path from these little localities to their sum' (2015a: 171). The complex forms can be divided into infinitely many straight-sided forms, but standard calculus settles for small enough, ignoring the infinitesimal remainder.

Hobbes wrote during the 'Age of Reason', a period marked by Descartes's invention of his method of certitude (Serres 1968a: 18n.1, 128, 132–133, 136; 2015a: 170–171). Hobbes, says Serres, only knows the state of war, a state of certainty (2015a: 163–164; 170–171). War eliminates uncertainty first by excluding foreign elements and then by standardizing the elements that remain, dressing them in uniforms and aligning them into grids, forming an orderly set, united against a clearly delineated common enemy. 'War is a homogeneous state' because it reduces individuals to resemblance, to uniformity, to elements unified into an ordered set (166–167). This standardization enables the Leviathan to 'integrate' the population, says Serres, using the vocabulary of integral calculus, replacing the organic notion of 'incorporation' with the mathematical notion of 'integration'. The orderly social body, the Leviathan, is formed by integrating standardised individuals. 'The big animal Leviathan was created by an integral calculus before its discovery; I would like to say that it makes this discovery possible', writes Serres in his chapter 'War and Plague' in *Rome*. Collectives, cities, and political states emerge from a process of standardization. 'Founding a city [like Rome] consists in standardizing the non-standard', he explains. The orderly state of war reduces the monads (which Leibniz defines as irreducible singularities) to resembling one another (171).

Conversely, in the non-standard state of plague, the monads lose their individuation but retain their irreducible singularity (171). Like the X in algebra, which designates the unknown quantity, the monad in a state of plague can take on any value. In contrast to the certainties of war, with its clear demarcation between friends and enemies, the state of plague, a state of uncertainty, is 'a possible state' because 'each individual takes on a thousand values' – friend, enemy, loved one, guest, host, and so on (168–169). Serres suggests that it may be possible to think about society using a non-standard model, as sets of elements without standardization. This will require, he says, 'a more subtle and broader new reason', as compared to the Leviathan's standardised reason (171). Under the conditions of the non-standard state, 'general hospitality doesn't chase anyone away; it's the feast without any excluded third' (179). The plague state, whether brought about by an actual epidemic or by another kind of social crisis, suggests the possibility of living in a state of general hospitality, leading Serres to ask,

> Can society, the social be thought otherwise than in sequential terms ...? Can we reason directly from the non-standard model, in disequilibrium

> and not in a state? Can we think without war, sets that would subsist without standardization? Utopia or new reason? A more subtle and broader new reason, suppler in any case, than the repetitive and slightly stupid rationality of the standard models. Will this new reason free us from the repugnant and ancient alliance of violence and war with our old reason? *(171–172)*

Serres accuses classical reason, exemplified by standard analysis, of exclusion and domination because it divides and discards infinitesimals while stripping monads of their singularity, reducing them to uniform elements. He dreams of replacing this 'repetitive and slightly stupid rationality' with a subtle, broad, and supple new reason, in the hopes of building a 'utopia' where humans live free from the old exclusionary reason allied with 'violence and war', the old reason which produced the military-industrial complex. These are the lessons Serres draws from the state of plague. The actual epidemic is not necessary for living a life of inclusive feasts, where all are invited and none are excluded. The open feast models a new social contract, under which humans live together, bound by the meal rather than by hostility toward a common enemy, as was the case with social bonds maintained in the state of war. In the plague state of general hospitality, 'The contract is the meal' (173).

Invisible Worlds

Mathematics is a field composed of multiple disciplines, several of which are practiced by Leibniz and Serres, who do not limit their application to mathematical objects (Serres 1968a: 66, 93–94). They acknowledge that mathematics works in mysterious ways, not always fully understood even by mathematicians. Rereading Camus's *The Plague*, sales of which have increased exponentially since the start of the Covid-19 pandemic, Jacqueline Rose observes that the novel's characters take comfort in the certitude of numbers, and yet 'Counting is at once a scientific endeavour and a form of magical thinking'. Numbers serve as 'a system for classifying the horror and bundling it away' (Rose 2020). Serres makes a similar observation in his reading of Musil's *The Man Without Qualities*. In modern society, death tends to be 'Quickly hidden, quickly carried off by the ambulance, quickly dissimulated in the jumble of statistics and in the calculation of the norm' (Serres 1978: 19). Like Camus's Doctor Rieux, every morning I consult the latest Covid-19 numbers, in search of certitude that the pandemic will end. I am seeking an omen presaging a miraculous decay in the slope of the curve, the lines of the graph that rise and fall, quantifying suffering and death, making the hidden viral enemy visible to me. For Serres, there exists 'a virtual world which is invisible, formal, and also multiply layered'. Mathematics and religion both provide access to this invisible world of abstraction (2019b: 9, 12, 20–32). Like the gods to whom humans offer sacrifices, feasts, and prayer, the *x–y* graph of mathematics – onto which the numbers of Covid-19 cases, hospitalizations, and deaths are plotted daily – only exist in realms beyond the physical world.

The invisible laws of mathematics explain the exponential spread of the virus throughout the social body. Sociologist Zeynep Tufekci explains the mathematics of SARS-CoV-2 contagion, illustrating the shocking difference in magnitude between a virus variant that infects an average of three other hosts versus one that averages four new infections:

> Increased transmissibility is an exponential threat. If a virus that could previously infect three people on average can now infect four, it looks like a small increase. Yet if you start with just two infected people in both scenarios, just 10 iterations later, the former will have caused about 40,000 cases while the latter will be more than 524,000, a nearly 13-fold difference.
>
> *(Tufekci 2021)*

The tiny virus quickly invades large-scale populations according to well-known mathematical formulas. Thanks to this law of propagation, a tiny entity threatens to decimate the species that otherwise dominates the planet. 'A small difference and there is unbelievable multiplication and uncountable destruction. Plague and flood. Endemic and epidemic diseases; variations of virulence, always small causes for either almost nonexistent or immense effects' (Serres 1982, 194).

Viewed through statistics, a collection of individuals becomes a population, an abstract social body. Curves on the *x–y* graph connect data points generated from objects in the world. These curves appear smooth and regular at the largest scales, even as at the smaller scales of virions and cells, random behaviour prevails, subject only to the laws of physical chaos (Serres 2006: 95–96, 184). As Serres puts it, 'Statistics plane down the variations proper to singular living things. The mathematical elimination of chance allows personal bodies to be known via a detour through the global'. These numbers do more than represent, when institutions and states rely on them to set policy and determine interventions. 'Nothing could be more effective than these calculations for mastering cures and administering the state of health of a numerous collectivity'. He notes that public health measures are often more effective than the more famous scientific discoveries (2019a: 24).

As mathematics professor Steven Strogatz observes, infinitesimals do not exist in the real world, but neither do other mathematical objects (2019: 203–204). However, the physical world operates in accordance to mathematical laws in ways that are still not entirely understood. Serres frequently references Galileo's pronouncement that nature speaks the language of mathematics and proclaims that the latter's greatest discovery was the interface between the virtual world and the physical world (2019b: 21–22). Humans have discovered how to intervene in the physical world by way of the virtual world of mathematics. With genetic engineering and the ever expanding powers of computing, nature's mathematical language has come to be understood in terms of code. 'All is code', remarks Serres, citing not only the genetic code but also alphabets, musical scales, databases, and money (2015b: 199–202; 2016: 163–167). Discussions of the coronavirus make frequent use of the language of codes – encoding, translating, transmission, transcription, expression (V'kovski et al. 2021). The 'messenger RNA' (mRNA) vaccines provide 'instructions' to cells to make harmless pieces of spike protein, telling them how to provoke an immune response (CDC 2021).

Feasts of the False Gods

Although virtual and invisible, encoding and mathematics produce real effects in the real physical world of existing bodies and things. In the realm of religion, the gods of ancient polytheism may no longer descend to earth, but 'false gods' do exist in the real world, and they thrive on a feast economy, with its lucrative hospitality sector. Continuous collective feasts take such forms as dining, entertainment, gaming, tourism, and the over-consumption of goods, a 'leisure economy' enabled by vast global transportation networks (Serres 2015b: 219–220). The current pandemic has been especially harsh on the precarious workforce that serves the new gods of the information age, those with the means to fully enjoy the modern feasts. The Roman logic of hospitality, which mandated opening the doors that won't protect us anyway, informs the contemporary pandemic strategy of opening bars, restaurants, hotels, and amusement parks, albeit more out of economic interest than in accord with the ancient laws of hospitality deconstructed by Derrida. This economic demand for a return to hospitality is accompanied by a desire to resume contemporary social rituals, such as birthday parties, weddings, funerals, worship services, family reunions, political rallies, concerts, spectator sports, and other large events. Quarantine has largely shut down these hospitable feasts, since all have become vectors for the respiratory virus that causes Covid-19. Many fear that the return of hospitality, enabled by vaccines, will reveal an even greater economic divide.

In *Angels: A Modern Myth*, Serres stages a dialogue between a scientific and a religious interpretation of the era of global travel. Pia, a doctor at the Charles de Gaulle airport in Paris, argues that the global information age divides the world vertically into two cities, one divine and the other mortal. Up above, local elites and the global bourgeoisie live in Newtown, connected by air travel, cell phone towers, and satellites, dwelling in gleaming towers or gated housing developments. This heavenly city, available to the few, occupies the abstract space of communication, finance, and distribution networks

(1995a: 69–74). However, this paradisiacal vertical city produces a hell below (72). Newtown, inhabited by the false gods of the information age, produces a 'global vertical disequilibrium' (170). Below, in Oldtown, dwell the workers who serve the false gods of Newtown. The two cities, Oldtown below and Newtown above, span the earth. Serres says that Oldtown 'is vaster in extent even than Newtown itself, and is integrally linked with it, except that it cannot hope to rise so high towards the stars' (75). Oldtown includes most of the third world, as well as the fourth world – the impoverished zones located within the first world. Says Serres:

> Oldtown – that great metropolis which is proliferating, chaotic, corrupt, dirty, sick, ragged, skeletal, anemic, and full of starving, corpselike babies – still regularly contributes to the upward mobility of Newtown, a very large amount of money, labour power, raw materials and human flesh.
>
> *(190)*

Serres explains the 'appalling inequality' between Newtown and Oldtown as a remnant archaic religion, resurrected as a new polytheism which divides the universe into heaven and hell, ancient social hierarchies reinterpreted as class struggle. The global economy has created false gods, who believe they earned their place in Newtown thanks to their skill or hard work, but whose antiseptic and overfed lifestyle is predicated on the poverty and labour of Oldtown, a legacy of previous regimes of exploitation. The workers of Oldtown feed the false gods of Newtown. Serres imagines Newtown as a modern-day Mount Olympus, where the new gods of the information economy engage in an endless feast, served by the inhabitants of Oldtown (191). As he puts it,

> the angels who soar in the upper reaches, and who drink complex pharmaceutical potions designed to keep death at bay, are today transformed into false gods, addicted to the Olympic banquet, in other words to an orgy of drugs and obesity. Ancient mythology provides a neat description of our current lifestyles.
>
> *(188–190)*

In the ancient feasts of the Olympic gods, Serres sees the archaic origins of current social hierarchies that shape populations, locally and globally. The poorest in the world lack access to the 'complex pharmaceutical potions' that enable the modern false gods to live longer with much better health. Hospitality encompasses not only better food, but better care and better medicine.

Hospitality and hospitals create profits on industrial and global scales, but while Oldtown produces hospitality and provides much of the hospital care, Newtown consumes most of it. As was the case with the great feasts for the gods on Mount Olympus, hospitality is still enjoyed disproportionately by the privileged. We live in a world of conditional hospitality, rather than in the utopia of general hospitality that Serres hopefully imagines. During time of plague, the Roman *lectisternia* may have opened the doors to all, but as Derrida explains, under the ancient Greek laws of hospitality, not everyone had the right to be welcomed as a guest, 'Because hospitality, in this situation, is not offered to an anonymous new arrival and someone who has neither name, nor patronym, nor family, nor social status, and who is therefore treated not as a foreigner but as another barbarian'. Without social credentials, the stranger or foreigner is an 'absolute other' receives no 'hospitality by right', contradicting the 'law of absolute hospitality' (2000: 23, 25). Global capitalism offers hospitality for a price, but no absolute hospitality. The new barbarians are simply the poor.

From Hotel to Hospital

Serres describes the plague as 'a strange bridge thrown from nature to culture. ... A strange passage from knowledge to a very archaic age', from modern science back to the earliest human societies. Modern knowledge explains epidemics and pandemics with virology and bacteriology, but these sciences do not explain the social and cultural behaviours and hierarchies that affect the course of infectious disease. This nature–culture bridge also spans the passage from hospitality to hospital, says Serres. 'This passage from the hotel to the hospital is the one I have named the Northwest Passage' (2015a: 172). The Northwest Passage across northern Canada figures, for Serres, the perilous pathways between the so-called hard sciences and the human sciences, the sciences of the world of things and the scientific study of social relations. The hotel, which can mean inn or private mansion in French, offers the lavish feasts of hospitality, while the modern hospital offers technologically advanced medical treatment. The poor of the world lack full access to either site.

In his later books, Serres recounts stories of human technological and social evolution, recognizing the mid-twentieth century as a turning point, marking a threshold between a period dominated by violent conflicts among the states of western Europe and a new period in which peaceful relations prevail. By this time, advances in science and medicine had doubled the human lifespan and allowed humans with access to healthcare to live relatively pain free, with enhanced pharmaceutical and surgical treatments that alleviate previously debilitating conditions. Describing this periodization, he identifies the era between the battle of Troy and the bombing of Hiroshima as the age of Napoleon the war hero, and declares the post-industrial era as the age of the Samaritan, who provided cared for a wounded stranger found on the side of the road. Military service, no longer obligatory in France, has given way to a 'politics of health', he suggests (2016: 102). His hope is that the science which produced the atom bombs dropped in 1945 will be rerouted toward the care and healing of humans, nonhumans, and the planet itself.

Alas, noting that healthcare remains as unevenly distributed as are the feasts, Serres laments that 'social injustice deprives the poorest of the benefits regarding pain and death'. Below in Oldtown, the mere 'mortals in pain' toil at precarious jobs, while 'the rare elect' feasting above in Newtown seek 'immortality'. For Serres, this social injustice is better understood through 'the history of myth, culture and religion' than through 'the history of science or even than history full stop'. Class difference has replaced 'the distance between the gods and humans'. In a modern pandemic, vaccines are ambrosia. Social injustice manifests itself in the obese bodies of the first world as compared to the emaciated bodies of the third world. 'Leaving ideology, politics becomes incarnated', writes Serres under the heading 'collective bodies' (2019a: 24–25).

Questioning the popular narrative that epidemics inspire violence, especially against foreigners, Cohn instead offers historical evidence that the far most common social response to epidemics is not hostility or violence, but care and compassion. Playing on the key phrase from Cohn's subtitle, 'Hate and Compassion', it could be said that societies tend to respond to plague with hospitality (compassion) rather than hostility (hate). However, during the present pandemic, there have been alarming incidents of aggression against Asians (targeted because Covid-19 is thought to have originated in China), as well as against those tasked with enforcing masking and distancing policies, such as retail workers, restaurant servers, and flight attendants. It is as if masking and distancing are perceived as inhospitable, if not hostile, a refusal of hospitality. As Covid-19 vaccinations begin to protect the wealthy while the poor continue to suffer and die in disproportionate numbers, the old tales of the ancient feasts of the immortals become more relevant than ever.

Notes

1 Travel and tourism are said to have accounted for more than 10% of the world economy in 2019 (Statista 2021).
2 *Leviathan* was published in 1651, when Leibniz and Newton, inventors of calculus, were still children.
3 For an online illustration, see Math is Fun.

References

Agamben, Giorgio. 2020. 'The Invention of an Epidemic' and 'Clarifications', in 'Coronavirus and Philosophers'. *The European Journal of Psychoanalysis*. https://www.journal-psychoanalysis.eu/coronavirus-and-philosophers/

Badiou, Alain. 2020, March 23. 'On the Epidemic Situation'. Translated by Alberto Toscano. *Verso* Blog. https://www.versobooks.com/blogs/4608-on-the-epidemic-situation

Castrillón, Fernando and Thomas Marchevsky (eds.). 2021. *Coronavirus, Psychoanalysis, and Philosophy: Conversations on Pandemics, Politics, and Society.* London: Routledge. https://doi.org/10.4324/9781003150497
CDC. 2021, March 4. 'Understanding MRNA COVID-19 Vaccines'. Centers for Disease Control and Prevention. https://www.cdc.gov/coronavirus/2019-ncov/vaccines/different-vaccines/mrna.html
Cohn Jr., Samuel. 2018. *Epidemics: Hate and Compassion from the Plague of Athens to AIDS.* Oxford: Oxford University Press. https://oxford.universitypressscholarship.com/view/10.1093/oso/9780198819660.001.0001/oso-9780198819660
Derrida, Jacques. 2000. 'Hostipitality'. Translated by Barry Stocker and Forbes Morlock. *Angelaki* 5(3): 3–18. https://doi.org/10.1080/09697250020034706
Derrida, Jacques and Anne Dufourmantelle. 2000. *Of Hospitality.* Translated by Rachel Bowlby. Stanford: Stanford University Press.
Esposito, Roberto. 2011. *Immunitas: The Protection and Negation of Life.* Translated by Zakiya Hanafi. Cambridge: Polity.
Math Is Fun. 2020. 'Introduction to Integration'. https://www.mathsisfun.com/calculus/integration-introduction.html
Peters, Michael A. 2020. 'Philosophy and Pandemic in the Postdigital Era: Foucault, Agamben, Žižek'. *Postdigital Science and Education*, 1–6. https://doi.org/10.1007/s42438-020-00117-4
Robinson, Abraham. 1996. *Non-Standard Analysis.* Princeton: Princeton University Press.
Rose, Jacqueline. 2020, May 7. 'Pointing the Finger'. *London Review of Books.* https://www.lrb.co.uk/the-paper/v42/n09/jacqueline-rose/pointing-the-finger
Serres, Michel. 1968a. *Le Système de Leibniz et Ses Modèles Mathématiques.* Paris: PUF.
Serres, Michel. 1968b. *Hermès I: La Communication.* Paris: minuit.
Serres, Michel. 1978. 'Exact and Human'. Translated by Winnie Woodhull and John Mowitt. *SubStance* 6(21): 9–19. https://doi.org/10.2307/3684460
Serres, Michel. 1982. *The Parasite.* Translated by Lawrence R. Schehr. Minneapolis: University of Minnesota Press.
Serres, Michel. 1983. *Hermes: Literature, Science, Philosophy*, Josué V. Harari and David Bell (eds.). Baltimore and London: The Johns Hopkins University Press.
Serres, Michel. 1995a. *Angels: A Modern Myth.* Translated by Francis Cowper. Paris: Flammarion.
Serres, Michel. 1995b. *The Natural Contract.* Translated by Elizabeth MacArthur and William Paulson. Ann Arbor: University of Michigan Press.
Serres, Michel. 1997. *Genesis.* Translated by Genevieve James and James Nielson. Ann Arbor: University of Michigan Press.
Serres, Michel. 2006. *Récits d'humanisme.* Paris: Pommier.
Serres, Michel. 2015a. *Rome: The First Book of Foundations.* Translated by Randolph Burks. London: Bloomsbury.
Serres, Michel. 2015b. *Le gaucher boiteux: Figures de la pensée.* Paris: Pommier.
Serres, Michel. 2016. *Darwin, Bonaparte et le Samaritain: Une philosophie de l'histoire.* Paris: Pommier.
Serres, Michel. 2019a. *Hominescence.* Translated by Randolph Burks. London: Bloomsbury.
Serres, Michel. 2019b. *Relire le relié.* Paris: Pommier.

Serres, Michel. 2020. *Branches: A Philosophy of Time, Event and Advent*. Translated by Randolph Burks. London: Bloomsbury.

Statista Research Department. 2021, February 4. 'Travel and Tourism: Share of GDP Worldwide 2000–2019'. https://www.statista.com/statistics/1099933/travel-and-tourism-share-of-gdp/

Strogatz, Steven. 2019. *Infinite Powers: How Calculus Reveals the Secrets of the Universe*. Boston: Houghton Mifflin Harcourt.

Toscano, Alberto. 2020. 'The State of the Pandemic'. *Historical Materialism* 28(4): 3–23. https://doi.org/10.1163/1569206x-12342804

Tufekci, Zeynep. 2021, May 28. 'Covid's Deadliest Phase May Be Here Soon'. *The New York Times*. https://www.nytimes.com/2021/05/28/opinion/covid-vaccine-variants.html

V'kovski, Philip, Annika Kratzel, Silvio Steiner, Hanspeter Stalder and Volker Thiel. 2021. 'Coronavirus Biology and Replication: Implications for SARS-CoV-2'. *Nature Reviews Microbiology* 19(3): 155–170. https://doi.org/10.1038/s41579-020-00468-6

Žižek, Slavoj. 2020. *Pandemic! COVID-19 Shakes the World*. Cambridge: Polity. Kindle edition.

INDEX

Pages in *italics* refer to figures and pages followed by "n" refer to notes.

FSC
www.fsc.org
MIX
Papier | Fördert
gute Waldnutzung
FSC® C083411

Kolibri 360 GmbH
Ferdinand-Jühlke-Straße 7
99095 Erfurt, Deutschland
produktsicherheit@kolibri360.de